CAMBRIDGE LIBRARY COLLECTION

Books of enduring scholarly value

History of Medicine

It is sobering to realise that as recently as the year in which On the Origin of Species was published, learned opinion was that diseases such as typhus and cholera were spread by a 'miasma', and suggestions that doctors should wash their hands before examining patients were greeted with mockery by the profession. The Cambridge Library Collection reissues milestone publications in the history of Western medicine as well as studies of other medical traditions. Its coverage ranges from Galen on anatomical procedures to Florence Nightingale's common-sense advice to nurses, and includes early research into genetics and mental health, colonial reports on tropical diseases, documents on public health and military medicine, and publications on spa culture and medicinal plants.

A Treatise on the Yellow Fever, as it Appeared in the Island of Dominica, in the Years 1793-4-5-6

In 1793, the Caribbean island of Dominica fell victim to the deadly yellow fever virus. The British physician James Clark (*c.*1737–1819), who practised on the island for many years, witnessed the outbreak at first hand. He published this descriptive account in 1797, using the work to discuss his methods of attempting to treat the disease, which was considered among the most lethal tropical ailments of the time. Long before the link between mosquitoes and disease transmission was made, Clark explains his hypothesis about the origins of the outbreak and discusses the symptoms of its sufferers as well as possible methods of prevention. He also includes chapters addressing other ailments, including typhus, dysentery, cholera and tetanus. This remains an enlightening resource in the history of the understanding and treatment of disease in tropical climates.

Cambridge University Press has long been a pioneer in the reissuing of out-of-print titles from its own backlist, producing digital reprints of books that are still sought after by scholars and students but could not be reprinted economically using traditional technology. The Cambridge Library Collection extends this activity to a wider range of books which are still of importance to researchers and professionals, either for the source material they contain, or as landmarks in the history of their academic discipline.

Drawing from the world-renowned collections in the Cambridge University Library and other partner libraries, and guided by the advice of experts in each subject area, Cambridge University Press is using state-of-the-art scanning machines in its own Printing House to capture the content of each book selected for inclusion. The files are processed to give a consistently clear, crisp image, and the books finished to the high quality standard for which the Press is recognised around the world. The latest print-on-demand technology ensures that the books will remain available indefinitely, and that orders for single or multiple copies can quickly be supplied.

The Cambridge Library Collection brings back to life books of enduring scholarly value (including out-of-copyright works originally issued by other publishers) across a wide range of disciplines in the humanities and social sciences and in science and technology.

A Treatise on the Yellow Fever,

as it Appeared in the Island of Dominica, in the Years 1793–4–5–6

To Which Are Added,
Observations on the Bilious Remittent Fever,
on Intermittents, Dysentery,
and Some Other West India Diseases

JAMES CLARK

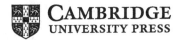

CAMBRIDGE
UNIVERSITY PRESS

CAMBRIDGE
UNIVERSITY PRESS

University Printing House, Cambridge, CB2 8BS, United Kingdom

Published in the United States of America by Cambridge University Press, New York

Cambridge University Press is part of the University of Cambridge.
It furthers the University's mission by disseminating knowledge in the pursuit of
education, learning and research at the highest international levels of excellence.

www.cambridge.org
Information on this title: www.cambridge.org/9781108065542

This edition first published 1797
This digitally printed version 2013

ISBN 978-1-108-06554-2 Paperback

A

TREATISE

ON THE

YELLOW FEVER,

AS IT APPEARED IN THE

ISLAND OF *DOMINICA*,

IN THE YEARS 1793-4-5-6:

TO WHICH ARE ADDED,

OBSERVATIONS

ON THE

BILIOUS REMITTENT FEVER,

ON

INTERMITTENTS, DYSENTERY,

AND SOME OTHER WEST INDIA DISEASES;

ALSO,

The CHEMICAL ANALYSIS and MEDICAL PROPERTIES

OF THE

HOT MINERAL WATERS

IN THE SAME ISLAND.

———————

BY

JAMES CLARK, M.D. F.R.S.E.

AND FELLOW OF THE COLLEGE OF PHYSICIANS OF
EDINBURGH.

PRINCIPIIS OBSTA.

LONDON:
Printed for J. MURRAY and S. HIGHLEY,
No 32, Fleet Street.

M. DCC. XCVII.

DEDICATION

TO

MAXWELL GARTHSHORE,

M.D. F.R.S. AND S.A.

AND

Member of the College of Phyficians of London, and F.R.S.
and College of Phyficians of Edinburgh, &c. &c.

SIR,

YOUR long and fteady Labours
for the Advancement of the
Practice of Phyfic in general, and
the great Attention you have fhewn
to Perfons employing their Time
for the Improvement of Medicine
in tropical Climates, encourage me
to addrefs to you the following
Treatife on the Yellow Fever, and

a 2   fome

DEDICATION.

fome other Difeafes of the Weft
Indies; and at the fame Time I
embrace the Opportunity of ac-
knowledging, in a public Manner,
the Obligations I owe to you for
your Politenefs and Friendfhip to
me on all Occafions.

I have the Honour to be, with great Efteem,

SIR,

Your much obliged
and very humble Servant,

JAMES CLARK.

London,
30th December 1796.

PREFACE.

THE following Obſervations on the Yellow Fever, which broke out in the Weſt Indies in the Year 1793, are ſolely founded on the experience I have been able to gain, during an extenſive practice in the iſland of Dominica.

With a view to avoid relating any thing which is not derived from my own experience and judgment, I have been cautious not to peruſe any of the publications which have appeared on the ſame ſubject: and I feel a ſatisfaction in affirming, that the care and attention I beſtowed on this diſeaſe for three years, whiiſt it raged with the moſt dreadful violence in all the Weſt India iſlands, have not been beſtowed in vain; the Method of Cure and Prevention here recommended, having been attended with very great ſucceſs during the above period.

The obſervations on the Bilious Remittent Fever, on Intermittents, Typhus Fe-

3   ver,

ver, Dyfentery, Dry Belly-ach, Cholera
Morbus, and the Tetanus, which follow in
this Work, are the refult of twenty-five
years conftant practice in the Weft Indies;
I therefore flatter myfelf that they will
prove ufeful to young and unexperienced
practitioners in that quarter.

I entertain the higheft opinion of the
merit and utility of the works of many of
the medical gentlemen, who have publifhed on thefe difeafes; but as in the former
cafe, I have avoided quoting or taking no-
tice of their practice, from the fame defire
to publifh only what has occurred to myfelf
in the hiftory and treatment of them, during fo long a refidence in that climate.

CONTENTS.

Chap. I.

Of the BILIOUS REMITTENT FEVER of the West Indies.

Chap. I.

Section

CONTENTS.

CHAPTER I.

SECTION I.

History of the YELLOW FEVER, *in the Island of Dominica.*

BY the prodigious influx of emigrants from the island of Martinique to the town of Roseau in this island, about the 10th June 1793, the streets and houses were very much crowded. The number of people that arrived here in the course of three days, to avoid the cruelty and persecution of their countrymen, could not be ascertained exactly, but it was estimated at between three and four thousand. These people were brought over in small vessels, exposed to the weather, and in want of almost every necessary of life. They were not sick on their arrival; and this fever had not made its appearance in Martinique when they left it, as many of the most respectable amongst them declared to me.

B   In

In a few days after their arrival, viz. the 15th June, this Fever first broke out; and the first victim to it was an English seafaring man, aged about forty, who had only been a fortnight on the island, and had never before been in the West Indies. Some days after, many of the sailors on board the ships in the Road were attacked; and then the unfortunate emigrants were the next sufferers. From the 1st July to the 1st October it was computed that eight hundred emigrants, including their servants and slaves, were cut off by this fever; and about two hundred English, including new-comers, sailors, soldiers, and negroes, also fell victims to it, in the same space of time. Few new-comers escaped an attack, and very few of these recovered. It spared neither age nor sex among the Europeans and emigrants who arrived; and not only the people of colour from the other islands, but the new negroes who had been lately imported from the coast of Africa, were all attacked with it. I knew a lot of twenty-four fine healthy new negroes all seized with this fever about the same time,

one

one third of whom died in the courfe of the difeafe. The negroes who had been long in the town, or on the ifland, efcaped; I only recollect one exception, which was in a negro who had undergone very great fatigue, and had been much expofed to the heat of the fun during a long journey.

Many emigrants fled from this ifland; but, alas! it was to fall a facrifice to the fame difeafe that now prevailed in every ifland. It appeared a few weeks earlier in Grenada and St. Vincent than it did in this, as we heard afterwards; and to the former it was fuppofed to have been brought by a Guinea fhip with negroes from the ifland of Bullam, on the coaft of Africa, and was therefore called the Bullam Fever. It was a few weeks later before it reached Antigua, and the reft of the Leeward Iflands; but all partook of its ravages during the autumnal months, and even till the month of December and January following.

During thefe months it alfo raged in Philadelphia; where, in the fpace of three months

only, four thoufand citizens were cut off
by it. It broke out about the fame time
at Jamaica and St. Domingo; from the latter
of which iflands the contagion was fuppofed
to have been brought to the town of Philadelphia.

This Fever became lefs violent here in the
month of October; and about the beginning
of November it ceafed altogether, which
was fuppofed to proceed from the comparative coolnefs of the weather; but the arrival
of fome American veffels, about fix weeks
after, convinced us that this fhort refpite was
more owing to the want of proper fubjects for
the vitiated atmofphere to act upon, than to
the change of its temperature; for in a fhort
time all on board, who had not been in the
Weft Indies before, were feized with it, and
although the mortality amongft them was
not fo great as it had been, yet many died.
This happened in December 1793, and January and February 1794. From this time
till the month of July few cafes occurred,
and moft of thefe recovered; and even in
the following autumnal months the mortality

tality was not near so great as in the former year.

After the 10th October 1794, when Berville camp in Guadaloupe surrendered, the emigration from that island commenced, and in a few weeks the town of Roseau was nearly as much crowded as it had been in June 1793. This fever did not appear among these people until the 10th of November, and although many of them died, it was by no means so fatal as before, nor did it last more than two months.

From the middle of January till July 1795 it disappeared; and even during this autumn only a few sailors, from irregularity of living, were attacked, and two cases only occurred in November: since which time to the 12th of June 1796, when I left the island, not a single case of this disease had occurred. The autumnal season, however, was then to be dreaded.

I find from my correspondents, that this fever has followed nearly the same course in all the leeward islands; only that it has been

rather

rather more violent, and continued longer,
in this, owing perhaps to the town being ſo
much crowded by the frequent emigration
of the French from the iſlands that were
ſituated near to us.

SECTION II.

The Symptoms.

THIS Fever ſometimes begins with a ſlight
rigor or chilly fit, rarely with ſhivering, ſuc-
ceeded by a violent head-ach and vomiting; but more frequently it comes on with
laſſitude, inclination to vomit, uneaſineſs
at the pit of the ſtomach, and a ſevere
pain in the back and forehead. The firſt
attack is generally in the night, or towards
morning; and very ſoon after, the eyes appear much inflamed, the face remarkably
fluſhed, and an uncommon redneſs about
the neck and breaſt ſucceeds. They cannot
bear the light; but turn their faces from it,
or cover their heads, and avoid it by every
means.

The

The fever comes on generally without any previous indifpofition, feizing the patient in a very fudden manner; but fome complained of laffitude and head-ach the day before. The pulfe feldom beats more than 90 in a minute; and the heat was never fo great as it is in the hot fit of an intermittent. The fick had not much defire for drink, and the tongue was not foul or white. What was vomited up during the firft twelve hours, was only the contents of the ftomach before, or what had been drank after the firft attack. Bile was feldom difcharged till eighteen or twenty-four hours after the firft feizure; but about that time or foon after, it became of a deep yellow colour, then green, and gradually darker, till at laft the black vomit made rts appearance; which happened in a few cafes as early as in thirty-fix hours, moft commonly in forty-eight, in fome not till the third or fourth day, and even as late as the fifth or fixth, although this occurred rarely,

The

The head-ach was of a peculiar kind, being intirely confined to the lower part of the forehead, the eye balls and their fockets. There was a remarkable inflammation in the tunica adnata, and flushing of the cheeks. An hœmorrhage from the nofe during the firſt twelve or eighteen hours feemed to relieve the head-ach, and fome recovered after this fymptom appeared; but if it did not come on before forty-eight or feventy-two hours, the difeafe proved fatal. Strong athletic people had generally fome degree of delirium during the febrile ſtage, and fome became quite outrageous. Women and delicate people were much dejected, and had a melancholic fort of delirium; but all were prepoffeffed with an idea of dying from the commencement of the difeafe. Their moſt uniform and conſtant complaint was want of ſleep; they never even dozed during this ſtage, as is ufual in other fevers. They all complained of pain and uneafinefs about the epigaſtric region; and frequently the liver feemed to be enlarged and hard, and preffing upon it occafioned confiderable pain.

Obſtinate

Obſtinate coſtiveneſs conſtantly prevailed,
and the common doſes of purgatives had no
effect whatever. The ſkin was generally dry,
and the heat of the body not much above
the natural ſtandard: the urine was not high
coloured as in the bilious remittent, or intermittent fevers, but after the febrile ſymptoms diſappeared it generally became yellow, or of a dark brown colour. The fluſhing of the face and the inflammation of the
tunica adnata began to abate before the yellowneſs about the neck appeared, this being the firſt part of the body that turned
yellow, and the eyes were ſoon after tinged.
Theſe appearances, together with an abatement of the febrile ſymptoms, finiſhed the
firſt or *febrile ſtage* of the diſeaſe.

As the life of the patient depends almoſt
entirely on the treatment during this ſtage
(for few have recovered if this was neglected
or ill treated) it is of the utmoſt conſequence
to pay attention to the moſt diſtinguiſhing or
true characteriſtic ſymptoms of this fatal diſeaſe. Theſe are chiefly, an extraordinary
fluſhing of the face, redneſs of the eyes, violent

lent pain in the eye-balls and round the lower part of the forehead, dry fkin, a full, foft pulfe, not much quicker than natural, and the heat, upon touching the body, found not to be fo great as the external appearances would lead us to expect.

For the firſt three months that this fever raged in Dominica, thefe were the fymptoms by which it was diftinguiſhed; but the following year it did not put on fuch remarkable diagnoſtic appearances. The fluſhing of the face, rednefs of the eyes, head-ach, &c. were lefs obfervable, and the feveriſh period was not fo foon over. They had no chillinefs on the firſt attack, the pulfe was full and foft, they had a flight delirium, the yellownefs did not appear before the fifth day, and many recovered.

There were a few exceptions to this account, but this was the ſtate of our patients in general; and the only difference from the fymptoms of the former year appeared to confiſt in the lefs degree of violence. An
4   hœmorrhage

hœmorrhage from the uterus often occurred, the menſtrual diſcharge was generally exceſſive, and was always a ſymptom of great danger.

About the cloſe of the febrile ſtage, there was often a violent hœmorrhage from the noſe, which was a bad ſign; as was a delirium firſt coming on at that time. In the ſpace of twelve hours after the yellowneſs of the neck, breaſt, and eyes came on, and the pulſe became ſlow, and the heat of the body natural, the black vomit made its appearance, unleſs a plentiful perſpiration had been brought on by medicine, and the vomiting put a ſtop to, or the mouth affeſted with mercury adminiſtered early in the diſeaſe.

This interval may be termed the *middle ſtage*. In ſome it was very ſhort, and then the diſeaſe proved fatal; if it was protraſted to the third day, and the vomiting ſubdued, the patient generally recovered. But to thoſe unacquainted with the diſeaſe, the ſymptoms at this period are very fallacious;

fallacious; the pulfe being quite flow, the heat of the body natural, the tongue clean, and fometimes moift; and if the patients are afked how they do? they will reply, very well. And as they cover their faces to avoid the light, a practitioner might be deceived if he did not inquire more into their real fituation, and uncover their faces; for from the peculiar appearance of the countenance much is to be learned in regard to life or death in this difeafe.

The bleeding at the nofe now became more violent, and was ftopped with great difficulty; the delirium and anxiety increafed, fome being quite outrageous, and others defpondent, muttering and moaning to themfelves; and fome having a placid, but unnatural fmile on their countenances, complaining from time to time of a pain about the epigaftric region, and vomiting foon after very dark yellow or green bile. In many, a fort of imperfect hiccup came on about this time; the prickly heat or mufquito bites on the body; and the elbows, from leaning on them in the

the act of vomiting, became of a scarlet
red colour, and the appearance of the true
skin on the removal of blisters was the
same. Some roared with a wild tone of
voice, shocking to the by-standers, fixing
their teeth, and refusing to take either drink
or nourishment.

Extreme restlesfsnefs and anguish generally precede the black vomit, which
may be styled the *putrefcent ftage* of the
difeafe. The hiccup becomes now more
evident, and the scarlet coloured fpots on
the skin and the parts that had been blif-
tered put on a pale purple hue. In fome,
blood iffued from the tongue; and the
hœmorrhage from the nofe, in thofe who
had had it before, increafed to a great degree, and contributed to fhorten the period
of the poor fufferer's life. What was vomited
up at this time, refembled grounds of
coffee, and feemed to be fmall particles of
black bile mixed with a ropy mucous fluid
and the contents of the ftomach.

The

The quantity of this black fluid, that was thrown up, is really aſtoniſhing. As the diſeaſe advanced, it became thicker and darker, till at laſt it reſembled the meconium of new born children ; the ſtools alſo became black, and had much the appearance and conſiſtence of tar. The hiccup became more violent and more frequent, and a total ſuppreſſion of urine came on. This ſymptom appears to proceed from a total ceſſation of the urinary ſecretion, as attempts have been made to draw off the urine by a catheter but without effect ; the bladder having been always found quite empty. If the urine had been paſſed in ſmall quantities at a time during the febrile ſtage, and tinged the linen yellow at the commencement of the ſecond, it was a bad ſign, and few that had this recovered. I never obſerved bloody urine ; and no blood was ever vomited up or paſſed by ſtool, except what ſeemed to have been ſwallowed by thoſe who had a violent bleeding from the noſe, which was not a conſtant ſymptom. After vomiting up a quantity of the black matter, the patients always ſeemed to

be

be relieved for a short period from that exceffive torture that they felt at the pit of the ftomach ; but on attempting to drink, the fame pain returned, and no liquid could then be retained for a moment on the ftomach. They had no difficulty of re-fpiration ; but great anxiety and oppreffion about the præcordia, and fometimes a tenfion over the epigaftric region, but rarely any diftention of the abdomen. After this the patient began to fink faft, the pulfe being now under 60 in a minute and the heat greatly below natural.

I never obferved cold clammy fweats in this difeafe, which happen fo often in the laft ftage of the bilious remittent fevers of thefe iflands, when they prove fatal. Nor have I ever obferved fubfultus tendinum, which is alfo fo common in the laft ftage of other fevers.

The debility was now fo great, that the pulfe often ceafed to beat, while the patient was vomiting, and the colour of the neck, arms, and legs became quite livid. Some were

were delirious at this time, but all were extremely reſtleſs, ſighing, and toſſing about,
till a general convulſion cloſed the diſtreſ-
ſing ſcene.   Theſe were the ſymptoms
amongſt young people; but the old and
infirm generally fell into a torpid comatoſe
ſtate, *after the febrile ſtage was over,* moaning and ſighing till they expired without a
ſtruggle.   This ſhocking ſtage of the diſeaſe
continued generally about twenty-four in
ſome thirty-ſix hours; but in others the progreſs of it was ſo rapid that the patient expired in a few hours after it began.

When the diſeaſe finiſhed its courſe in
ſeventy-two hours, the different ſtages followed one another in ſuch a rapid manner,
that it was ſcarcely poſſible to diſtinguiſh
them.   It was protracted in general to the
fifth day, in ſome to the ſeventh, and in a
few inſtances to the eighth or ninth, before
death took place.   In one patient the
yellowneſs continued till the thirteenth day,
and as he retained medicines and nouriſhment on his ſtomach, and a number of
boils

boils broke out on his face, head, and neck, we entertained hopes of his recovery; but the nurſe having neglected to adminiſter bark and nouriſhing cordials as directed, ſome of theſe boils became gangrenous, and he expired in a convulſion the fifteenth day of the diſeaſe.—In many this putrid tendency was ſo far advanced, before we were called to the ſick, that no medicine or any application whatever .ſeemed to have any power or effect in checking its progreſs towards a total diſſolution.

SECTION III.

The Prognoſtic.

WHEN the practitioner was not called in during the febrile ſtage, or until the black-vomit and other putrid ſymptoms had appeared, which happened to be too often the caſe, it was no difficult matter to pronounce with certainty the fatal event of the diſeaſe.—In general few recovered who had a *cold* fit at the beginning of the fever.

If the yellowneſs appeared in twenty-four

C or

or thirty-fix hours after the firft attack, when the cafe had been left to nature, or the patients had been bled, and no powerful remedies attempted, they never recovered.—Or whether the yellownefs appeared or not, if the fever left great languor and debility, there was no expectation of a recovery.—The fooner the febrile ftage ended, when the cafe was left to nature, or only fimple remedies were ufed, the greater the danger; and, on the contrary, the fooner the fever was fubdued by powerful remedies acting in an evident and decifive manner, the greater chance the patient had to recover.—If the debility was not great after the fever, and the yellownefs did not appear before the fourth or fifth day, the fick generally recovered.—Many alfo recovered after the yellownefs, and even after a violent bleeding at the nofe had begun; but in all my practice I only recollect four patients who recovered after the black vomit had made its appearance.

None recovered after a violent hiccup came on, or a total fuppreffion of urine.

Children,

Children, adults, and old people labouring under the fmall-pox were conftantly
attacked with this fever. about the time
that the fecondary fever ufually comes on,
and none recovered, but thofe who had
begun to take bark and wine after the
eruptive fever, and continued this remedy
and a nourifhing diet for fome time after.
It made no difference whether the fmall-
pox were of the confluent or diftinct benign
kind.—All fell victims to this difeafe, who
were not treated in the manner mentioned
above.—Thofe who recovered of this fever
were never attacked a fecond time, at leaft
no inftance occurred of it in our ifland,
nor in any of the other iflands, as far as I
have been informed.—Neither were they
fubject to be attacked with an intermittent, as thofe who had recovered from the
bilious remittent fever of the Weft Indies in
general are; but they had a very long convalefcence.

On diffection, a great quantity of the
fame kind of black vifcous fluid was found
in the ftomach, that had been vomited up

C 2　　　　　　　before

before death.—The gall bladder and the
ducts were filled with black bile, of a ropy
viscid consistence, and the liver seemed to
be enlarged and *soft*, but not otherways
apparently diseased; the spleen did not seem
to be much affected.—The intestinal canal
was filled with a viscid black stuff, of a
thicker consistence than that which was
found in the stomach, and very much re-
sembled tar, or very thick meconium."

The cadaverous offensive smell of those
in a dying state or directly after death, did
not appear to me to be so considerable, as
it is in those dying of the bilious remittent
fever; but the body turned quite black
very soon after death.

SECTION IV.

THE French call this fever the Maladie
de Siam, for the same reason that it
is termed the Bullam fever in Grenada;
and sometimes it is also called Maladie des
Matelots, on account of sailors being particularly

ticularly liable to it.—The Spaniards call it Vomito-nigro, from the black vomit which never fails to make its appearance towards the clofe of the difeafe; but it is of little ufe to know this diftinguifhing fymptom at fo late a period. It appears to be a fever of the typhus kind, and very properly called typhus icterodes in Dr. Cullen's fynopfis.—Perhaps the heat (as it is only in very hot weather, or in very hot climates that it appears) occafions that great determination of fluids to the liver, and that extraordinary fecretion of vitiated bile, which characterizes this from all other fevers of the typhus kind, and renders it more fatal than any other, the plague not excepted.—I think the term Yellow Fever the beft adapted to diftinguifh it from others, and I have therefore continued it.

I have never feen any publication on this fever fince it broke out in the Weft Indies and America in the year 1793; but I had letters frequently on this fubject from my worthy friend Dr. Wright of Edinburgh, now phyfician to his majefty's

forces

forces in Barbadoes, and I communicated to him from time to time my obfervations on this difeafe, and the fuccefs of my method of cure. I have been informed that it has been confidered, by fome authors, as an imported and very infectious difeafe; but in this ifland it did not appear to be either imported or infectious. The very few inftances which feemed to indicate contagion, I think may be accounted for on other principles.—Some inhabitants who had been accuftomed to breathe a cool healthy air in high fituations in the country, were fometimes attacked after a vifit to town, in the fame manner as new-comers from Europe and America, who never had been in the Weft Indies before; the reafon of which will be inquired into hereafter.—Thofe who had refided long in town, or near the fea-fide, were not attacked with it.—The phyficians and furgeons who vifited the fick, and the nurfes who attended them conftantly, were not infected, nor did there occur a fingle inftance of one of them being feized with this fever for thefe three years that I have remained in the ifland, fince it broke out; altho' no prophylactic, or precaution of any

fort

fort whatever, was made ufe of to counter-
act or avoid contagion. I am therefore of
opinion, that this terrible difeafe was not imported into this or any other of thefe iflands,
or into America, but that it was produced
from natural caufes. I do not contend,
however, that it did not become contagious
in fome meafure afterwards, in fome of the
towns, fhips, or other places, in proportion
to the degree of concentration of the vitiated
air in them, both in this climate and in
America. But I fhall poftpone my enquiry
into the remote caufes of this fever, until
I have treated fully on the method of cure,
which is by far the moft important part of
my fubject, and ought to be particularly
attended to.

SECTION V.

Method of Cure.

THE firft indication is to fubdue the
fever by the moft fpeedy means in our
power. The fecond is to prevent the putrefcent ftate that follows fo rapidly after the

C 4   febrile

febrile ftage, or to oppofe its progrefs when
begun, and at the fame time to fupport the
ftrength of the patient.   From the remarkable flufhing of the face, great inflammation
of the eyes, and full pulfe in the firft ftage
of this difeafe, young practitioners might
be induced to ufe the lancet freely, and the
French furgeons, whofe chief remedy in almoft all diforders in thefe iflands is venefection, very readily fell into this error.   There
was not a fingle inftance of an emigrant recovering who had been bled.   The Englifh
practitioners avoided bleeding their patients,
and very few of the French, who put themfelves under their care from the beginning
of the difeafe, died of it.   Some time after
a few cafes occurred that feemed to require
bleeding, and it was employed with fuccefs;
but thefe were new-comers immediately
from Europe, who had never been in the
Weft Indies, of a robuft make, and fanguine
temperament.   A pound, and in fome two
pounds of blood were taken away early in
the difeafe, with feeming advantage, and
fome recovered who were treated in this way;
but it failed of fuccefs in others, and at laft it
was

was laid aside altogether. It should be observed, that we were seldom called in time
to make use of venesection with advantage,
even when a proper subject offered. In
young athletic people, seized with this
fever soon after their arrival in the West
Indies, venesection to a certain degree may
be of use, if performed during the first
twenty-four hours from the attack, but if
used after that period, or at most after
thirty-six hours, it will always be found
prejudicial, if not fatal. It ought to be laid
down as a general rule, never to bleed the
natives of the West Indies, nor those from
Europe, who by residence for a certain
time have lost the inflammatory deathesis
in their blood, or in other words are seasoned to the climate. Nor should the officers
of the navy or army, or their men, when
seized with this fever, after having undergone excessive fatigue, and exposure to the
violent heat of the sun in a hard campaign,
ever be bled. This rule is founded on experience; and the reason is obvious.

                              Pediluvium

Pediluvium and a purging clyfter were generally firft ordered, to moderate the violent determination to the head, while more powerful remedies were preparing. Purging was the chief means employed to remove the fever, but the ftomach could feldom be brought to retain the common purgatives: and even when they were not vomited up, a triple dofe was always neceffary to procure fufficient evacuations by ftool. Two drams of jalap were often adminiftered by degrees, and although all retained on the ftomach, this large quantity failed to operate fufficiently, and the little effect it produced was not till fix or eight hours after it had been taken, whereby much time, which is fo very precious in this difeafe, was loft. From frequent difappointments in this way, I was led to add calomel to the jalap, which was ordered to be made up in the following form:

℞ Pulv. jalapii. ℈ij.
    Calomelan. pp^{ti} ℈j.
    Ol. menthæ guttas iv.
    Aquæ fontanæ. q. s. fiat maffa
      in pilulas xvi dividenda.

                              Of

Of thefe pills fix or eight were given as
fpeedily as poffible, with a cup full of cold
mint or cinnamon tea, and two or three
more repeated every hour till they operated. If they were thrown up, which fometimes happened, ten grains of calomel were
formed into two pills, which were adminiftered immediately, and repeated in four
hours, if they had not operated plentifully
before that time. The patients were allowed mint, bafil, or cinnamon tea, or, in
fhort, whatever weak diluents they relifhed
moft, for their common drink, except cold
water; but they were always enjoined to
drink very little at a time. Crem. tartar
whey was very grateful to the fick, and was
often ufed. After the purgative was fuppofed to have operated fufficiently, if the
head-ach was not relieved, a blifter was applied to the neck, or over the occiput; and
a perfpiration was encouraged, by giving
warm drinks when the vomiting was not
very violent; three or four grains of calomel
were given, in a pill, every four or fix hours,
to which fometimes opium was added,
                                    when

when the purging had a tendency to run to
excefs; in the following form:

℞ Calomelan. pp'' Əi.
   Opii puri g'ᵃ iv.
   Olii cinnamomi guttas iv
   Aquæ fontanæ. q. s. fiat in pilulas
   N° vi. capiat unam omni quarta
   vel fexta hora.

The ufe of thefe pills was continued during
the whole of the febrile ftage, and often for
fome days after.—Thefe medicines feldom
failed to remove the fever in twenty-four
or thirty-fix hours, if the vomiting was not
fo violent, that neither medicines nor drinks
could be retained on the ftomach, which
fometimes happened.—In this cafe a blifter
was applied over the epigaftric region,
which generally checked the vomiting, and
had a good effect when employed early in
the difeafe. I found that bliftering any
other parts of the body than thofe mentioned above, anfwered no good purpofe;
that it ferved only to torture the patient,
and was even frequently hurtful. Bliftering

ing was seldom employed, except when the
vomiting could not be stopped otherwise,
and never used after the febrile stage of
the disease.   This was the result of experience, for at first we tried them in the
second stage, and found they answered no
good purpose.   When there was very little
or no inclination to vomit, I added pulvis
antimonialis to the calomel, in the following form :

> ℞ Pulver. antimonialis ℈i.
> Calomelanos pp^{ti} g^{ra} x.
> Syrupi simplicis. q.s. fiat. massa
> in pilulas viij dividenda *.

Four of these pills were immediately given,
and two more repeated every second or
third hour after, till they had some effect.
If the first four occasioned a reaching or
vomiting, no more were given, and the calomel pills were resorted to.   A grain or
two of opium was given afterwards, to settle

* Sometimes equal quantities of the antimonial powder and calomel were made up, and divided into the
same number of pills; and sometimes James's powder
was used in the same way.

the

the ftomach and to procure fleep. If this medicine operated plentifully by ftool before the opiate was adminiftered, and a profufe perfpiration followed, the fever was carried off in twenty-four hours, and the patient recovered; notwithftanding which, the calomel pills were continued, and the antifeptic plan purfued for feveral days after. When the calomel alone, or joined to the antimonial, operated very powerfully, chicken broth, and panada, or fago with Madeira wine or old hock, was ordered to fupport the patient, and fometimes it was found neceffary to order an anodyne draught to moderate the operation of thefe powerful remedies. The antimonial or James's powder, when joined to calomel, rarely occafioned vomiting. Their effects were, commonly, to excite perfpiration and procure a few ftools. This preparation, however, was not ufed fo often as calomel alone, or with jalap. The vomiting was fo much dreaded, that we chofe to truft to thefe rather than run the rifk of increafing or exciting this too often fatal fymptom, by an antimonial of any kind; yet the antimonial thus

combined

combined had a very good effect upon some,
when administered very early in the disease;
and in all cases which are looked upon as
very desperate, it ought to be tried. The
dose of the antimonial, and also of calomel,
when used as an evacuant, may appear to
be too large, and even dangerous: but to
this most desperate of all diseases, it is necessary to oppose, very speedily, the most
powerful, and even seemingly desperate remedies *. The effects of them were, however, generally restrained by opium, as before mentioned, when their operation, either
upwards or downwards, tended to weaken
the patient. None of the French, who were
treated in a trifling manner by their own
surgeons in this island, ever recovered.
Some indeed were hastened to their graves
by frequent bleedings and the warm bath.
Others were lost for want of active purgatives at the commencement of the disease;
their cure having been, in general, trusted

* Hippocratis Aphorism. Sectio i. Aphorism 6.

to

to clyfters, ptifans, and a dofe of manna, or crem. tartar.

After the febrile ftage, the calomel was continued to be given as an alterative, in dofes proportioned to the apparent danger, with or without opium, according to the ftate of the primæ viæ. From three to four grains of calomel in the form before mentioned, were adminiftered every four or fix hours to an adult, and a glafs of ftrong decoction or infufion of red bark with orange peel, was ordered every hour and a half in the intervals, together with as much nourifhment and wine as the ftomach could bear, but always given in fmall quantities, and often repeated. In this way we proceeded for thirty-fix or forty-eight hours after the febrile ftage was over, by which time the fate of the patient in general might be determined; other more fimple means were fometimes employed, to oppofe the fuppofed putrid tendency in the fluids, as will be hereafter mentioned. A ptyalifm rarely took place, but the gums were fometimes a little affected about the third day, in which cafe the mercury and

every

every other remedy was fufpended, and nourifhment and wine only given; when this happened we could venture to prognof-ticate, with confidence, the recovery of our patients. But it was too frequently the cafe, that we were not called to the fick till the middle ftage, when the yellownefs had ap-peared. At this time we had to combat with great languor and debility, attended with great uneafinefs at the ftomach, and a conftant reaching to vomit.

If a purgative had not been adminiftered before, a purging clyfter was ordered, and three or four graius of calomel given every five or fix hours with or without opium, according to the patient's ftrength; the above antifeptic plan purfued, and nourifh-ment and wine given frequently. If they had been purged, an opiate with calomel or an anodyne draught was ordered, and the alterative pills, and the decoction of bark, &c. given as to thofe who had been under our care from the beginning. At firft, as has been before obferved, we tried a blifter over the epigaftric region, but finding it an-

D   fwered

fwered no good purpofe at this period of the difeafe, it was not continued afterwards. Epithems of aromatic herbs, fpices, muf- tard, and wine, &c. were applied over the region of the ftomach to check the reach- ing, but to little purpofe. Bark in fub- ftance never would fit on the ftomach. The ftrong decoction of the red bark, to which the fpiritus ætheris vitriolici was added, ge- nerally remained on the ftomach, and agreed better than the common bark. A fmall tea-fpoonful of this vitriolic æther was given in four table-fpoonfuls of this decoction every hour and a half, or two hours. Some- times this vitriolic æther was given in ftrong camomile or fnake-root tea, when the bark was rejected ; and when neither of thefe would remain upon the ftomach, it was given in peppermint-water, or plain water and fugar, or in what is called fan- gree ; and in general it proved very cordial to the fick, and grateful to the palate. Clyfters of the decoction of bark with this fpirit, or with vinegar or lime-juice, were thrown up every two or three hours; and fometimes the body was rubbed over with

lime-

lime-juice or vinegar. The ftrained juice
of the oxalis, or wood-forrel, was given in-
wardly, and ufed in clyfters, with more
evident good effects, in reftraining the
putrid tendency, than any other acid. I
knew two patients, who had only taken a
few calomel pills, and afterwards by the
ufe of this acid, with wine and nourifhment, recovered, after the fecond ftage had
made great progrefs, and even after the
black-vomit had appeared in one of them,
without any other remedy whatever. Elixir
of vitriol was tried, but the mineral acids
were not found to fit fo eafily on the ftomach as the vegetable. A glafs of peppermint-water, from time to time, relieved the
uneafinefs at the pit of the ftomach, or a
few drops of the effence was given on a
bit of fugar. When a bleeding from the
nofe came on, alum-whey was given for
common drink, and the hœmorrhage was
reftrained by a ftrong folution of white vitriol. Great attention was paid to cleanli-
nefs in the houfes or fhips where the fick
lay, and vinegar was fprinkled frequently
all over them every day. Branches of
D 2   fhrubs

ſhrubs and leaves of trees were ſprinkled with water, and ſometimes with vinegar and water, and put in the windows where the rays of the ſun came, in order to aſſiſt in purifying the air of the rooms by increaſing the quantity of vital air.   Vinegar was frequently thrown on hot iron in the chambers of the ſick, with the ſame intention. All this time wine was adminiſtered gradually, either with water and ſome grateful acid, or mulled with ſpices, as the ſtate of the patient required.   Pure æther was of little ſervice, the effects of it being ſo ſoon over.   Camphor ſeemed to ruffle the ſtomach, and increaſe its irritability, and was laid aſide after a few trials.   Muſk had no effect whatever on the hiccup, and being an expenſive remedy, was, after ſix or eight trials, left off.   Opium procured ſome reſpite from this ſymptom.   Saline draughts, given in the act of efferveſcence, checked the vomiting for a time, and were really ſerviceable, eſpecially in the firſt ſtage of the diſeaſe.   But all theſe means and ſimpler remedies were ineffectual to reſiſt the fatal tendency of the diſeaſe, and were only conſidered fidered by us in the light of collateral aids. Our greateft dependance, or, in the nautical ftyle, our fheet-anchor, was mercury. Antifeptics, tonics, wine, and nourifhment, were no doubt alfo abfolutely neceffary, and without which, perhaps, this remedy would have failed of fuccefs.

I was led to the ufe of calomel in the firft ftage, on account of the tardy and ineffectual operation of other purgatives, as before mentioned. At that period, the neceffity of purging feemed to be clearly pointed out, from the evidently violent determination of the circulation to the head. In the fecond ftage, the determination appeared to be equally violent to the liver, which was then the principal feat of the difeafe.

Mercury is known to remove in an extraordinary manner, the principal difeafes of the liver, fuch as the chronic hepatitis, and obftructions from repeated and long continued attacks of intermittents, and to correct a vitiated or fuperabundant fecretion of bile, and alfo to cure the dyfentery fup-

D 3   pofed

poſed to proceed from thence; all which
no other medicine yet diſcovered, is poſ-
ſeſſed of ſuch power to effect: And as every
indiſpoſition or complaint ariſing from an
over ſecretion of bile, ſo common in the
Weſt Indies, is moſt ſpeedily and effectually
removed by calomel, employed as an alterative as well as a purgative, I was induced by analogy to continue the uſe of
mercury with this intention, after the febrile ſtage was over, and it has fully an-
ſwered my expectation. In a few caſes of
this fever, where there was an evident en-
largement of the liver, and where the inceſſant vomiting prevented our throwing in
a ſufficient quantity of calomel in a ſhort
time, I uſed frictions of ſtrong mercurial
ointment over the hypochondria and epigaſtric region. If the gums were affected
by the rubbing, all went on well. But this
method of cure was not ſufficiently purſued,
owing to the trouble that it gave to the
nurſes. I think it a good practice in all
caſes where we are much preſſed for time,
or ſuch as are conſidered to be very deſperate. In hoſpitals it ought to be attempted,
                                    eſpecially

especially on such patients as can scarcely retain medicine or drink on their stomach for a moment, which happens very often, and these are always looked upon as truly desperate cases. After the black-vomit has made its appearance, there is little to be hoped from any remedy. But to shew the powers of mercurial friction, I cannot but add, that in two cases of idiopathic tetanus; I ordered a pound of mercurial ointment to be applied by friction to each, in he course of three days, by which the gums were affected, the spasms abated, and both patients speedily recovered. The dry belly-ach, which is also a violent spasmodic malady, is likewise cured by mercurial frictions, as well as by calomel; for this disease is removed as soon as the mercury affects the mouth, which happens generally before stools are procured ; and even when a plentiful alvine evacuation takes place, the symptoms are seldom if ever removed entirely, till the mercury takes effect. In short, I am convinced from long experience, that mercury is fully as useful, and as indispensably necessary for the cure of all

D 4   diseases

diseases of the bilious and spasmodic kind between the tropics, as the Peruvian bark is in the remittent and intermittent fevers of all warm climates. Without the aid of these two invaluable remedies, perhaps few Europeans who visit hot climates, would live to return to their native land. I tried the sea-water bath on some patients, who could not retain medicine. A large pailful or two of cold salt water was thrown over them four times a day, and after being well dried, they were covered, and had some warm mulled wine or sangree given to them. This seemed to have a good effect for a short time, and it appeared to retard the progress of the disease; but it did not, upon the whole, succeed well in this Island; probably from its having been in general tried when too late; for my friend Dr. Archbald of the island of Nevis, certainly employed this method of cure often with success; and I have heard that it has also succeeded sometimes in Jamaica. It ought to be used after a purging clyster, or after a purgative, but not after mercury has been administered. Our confidence in mercury,

prevented

prevented our making more frequent trials of sea-bathing, as the use of both at the same time we conceived to be incompatible.

When called early in the second stage of the disease, we found that by the use of mercury, a steady perseverance in the antiseptic plan, good nursing and care, many of our patients recovered, and some even after the black-vomit came on, as was mentioned before, in whom however the other mortal symptoms, such as violent hœmorrhage from the nose, hiccup, and suppression of urine, were wanting.

But in the worst cases, or such as had been neglected at the beginning, where the septic process had got such a firm hold of the system, that it proceeded with a gradual but steady step, increasing in violence every hour, till at last a total dissolution of the whole system took place, no remedy that we tried seemed to have any power even to retard, much less to resist its fatal progress.

From

From a firm belief that this difeafe was by
no means contagious in our ifland, the fick
were not abandoned by their friends, nor
negleƈted by their attendants, which contributed very much to the recovery of
many who would otherwife have been loft
for want of care. When the opinions of
medical gentlemen, who praƈtife phyfic in
the Weft Indies or America, lean to the fide
of this being a very infeƈtious difeafe, it is of
the utmoft confequence to conceal them as
much as poffible from the attendants on
the fick, and even to hold out a contrary
opinion, for otherwife the fick will be
abandoned to their fate ; and the dread of
infeƈtion will operate fo powerfully on the
minds of the people, that many will be
feized with the difeafe when it becomes
more frequent, and the air is farther vitiated,
who, if not influenced in this manner,
might have efcaped an attack. A ftrong
confidence in fome, that a difeafe is not infeƈtious, and a great fortitude of mind in
others, who conceive it to be fo, or their
firm reliance on fome favourite plan of pre-

vention, are perhaps the greateſt preſerva-
tives * we know againſt any contagion.

* When I make uſe of the plural "we," I mean my
friend Dr. Fillan of Dominica, who had an equal ſhare
of the buſineſs with myſelf, and of courſe followed the
ſame method of practice,

CHAP.

CHAPTER II.

SECTION I.

The Method of Prevention.

W H E N the difeafe was become frequent
and raged with violence, many new-comers
from Europe were attacked with it in eight
or nine days after their arrival ; fome were
feized a fortnight after, of thefe I knew
three young men from 13 to 15 years of age,
who arrived the fame day on the ifland, and
were attacked that day fortnight all about
the fame hour, one of whom died the fifth
day, and the other two recovered; but of
thefe I only attended one, who was cured
by mercury. Many were not feized till
after a month or fix weeks refidence; and
I remember one inftance of a perfon dying
of this difeafe, after he had been nine
months in the Weft Indies, and had vifited
other iflands. But, in general, the attack
upon new-comers was during the firft
month

month or fix weeks after their arrival.
Officers of the navy and army were rarely
attacked during the fevere fatigues of a
campaign, and even when expofed to the
violent heat of the fun; but in a few weeks
after they were relieved from it, and repofe
fucceeded to exceffive exertion and anxiety
of mind, very few efcaped an attack. Emigrants who had endured much fatigue in
their flight, had lived on poor nourifhment,
had bad lodging and little fleep, and who
had been haraffed by the influence of fear,
grief, and exceffive heat, all of which are
powerful pre-difpofing caufes, were attacked almoft to a certainty in a week or ten
days after. When this fever prevails, I
found one bleeding neceffary for new comers of a fanguine temperament and a robuft
make, and a cooling purgative the next day;
and ordered them to live chiefly on a vegetable diet and fruits, and to avoid the heat
of the fun as much as poffible, and to take
fome cooling laxative medicine frequently
during the firft month or fix weeks. But
lately my chief dependance was on mercury.
A purge of calomel and jalap was firft
                                        given,

given, and frequently repeated, or a few grains of calomel were given once or twice a day till the gums were affected, and a purgative afterwards; and soon after, this course was renewed without confining the patient, and after this some bark was generally ordered every day for a week or more. Few could be prevailed upon to continue the mercurial course long enough, and fewer ftill to renew it, but such as did were not attacked. On the arrival of Europeans, a few calomel purges in the course of the firft ten days, with a vegetable diet, and the moderate use of wine, together with bark for several days after, and the renewal of the calomel purges and bark from time to time during the firft two or three months residence, was the moft common method employed to prevent an attack, and it was generally fuccefsful. It is worthy of remarking, however, that a ftrong dose of calomel was commonly given upon the leaft indifposition, or appearance of an attack, and bark in infusion or otherwise taken for some days after. The officers of his Majefty's navy and army, who have leisure and can

be

be prevailed upon, on their arrival, to un-
dergo one or two gentle courfes of mercury,
taking a few laxative medicines after, confining themfelves to the moderate ufe of
wine, and living chiefly on vegetables and
fruits for the firft two months, may rely
almoft to a certainty on efcaping this fever.
But if the nature of the fervice requires
their exertions immediately, which has generally been the cafe fince this fever firft
broke out, a few brifk calomel purges as
foon as poffible after their arrival, and bark
at intervals during the fervice that they may
be upon, will generally fecure them againft
an attack.   But as foon as the fervice is
over, they ought then to be moft attentive
to prevent an attack, and not to neglect, if
poffible, taking calomel for feveral days,
and bark afterwards. The fame plan ought
to be followed in regard to the failors and
troops in thefe iflands, but this muft be attended with much difficulty, and I fhall not
prefume to advife the medical gentlemen of
the navy and army on this head.   Their
own experience has no doubt pointed out
to them the readieft and fafeft mode of ad-
ministering

miniftering medicines, and alfo the beft method of treatment; my intention here being only to recommend, in the ftrongeft manner, the liberal ufe of mercury when an opportunity offers, both as a prefervative againft, as well as an effectual remedy for this fever; and in the former cafe, to fortify the conftitution by the plentiful exhibition of bark, continued for fome time. efpecially after a. hard campaign, or great fatigue and expofure to the exceffive. heat of the fun. The emigrants could not bear much purging; one döfe of calomel and rhubarb was fufficient for them, and bark afterwards, renewing the purgative occafionally. This method fecured all againft an attack, who were under our care in this ifland. Some new comers, who efcaped this fever by the means above-mentioned, had fome months afterwards an attack of the remittent bilious fever, or of an intermittent, neither of which are dangerous difeafes when attended to in the beginning, being confidered here as only a feafoning to the climate.

CHAP-

CHAPTER III.

SECTION I.

An Inquiry into the remote Causes of this Fever, at Dominica, and in the other Islands, and in North America.

1st. DURING the hurricane months of the year 1792, there was very little thunder in this island, and the weather was very sultry. From the month of January to the 15th of June 1793, when this fever first broke out, the weather was extremely calm, and much hotter than usual in this, as well as the neighbouring islands. There was little rain till the 15th of October.

2d. We had no thunder in the months of May and June, nor in the autumn of the year 1793, which had not been the case here for twenty years before. This circum-

E   stance

ſtance was alſo remarked in the other iſlands.

3d. Fahrenheit's thermometer, in the months of June, July, Auguſt, and September of the ſame year, generally roſe to 88 or 90 degrees, and ſometimes to 92°, between the hours of two and four o'clock, P. M. when placed in a large room, with all the doors and windows left open to admit freſh air, as is cuſtomary in the Weſt Indies. At ten o'clock at night it ſeldom fell below 80°, and at daylight in the morning, which is the coldeſt time of the twenty-four hours, 79 degrees was the loweſt. When the thermometer was carried about in the ſtreets of the town, it roſe to 110 degrees ; and when hung up in the ſun, the mercury was ſoon at 120°.

In former years the thermometer had been frequently obſerved to riſe to 90 and even to 92 degrees, in the autumnal months ; but it never continued long at this height ; for the cloudy weather, heavy rains, and

a   thunder

thunder ftorms, which never failed to happen at that feafon, cooled the atmofphere.
The heat, for fome months before, and during the continuance of this fever in the
ifland, efpecially in the night-time, was almoft 'infupportable. The variation in the
rife or fall of the mercury in the barometer
in thefe iflands is fo little, that keeping an
account of it did not appear to me to be of
confequence.

4thly. I was informed by a gentleman,
who was in North America when this fever
broke out at Philadelphia, that there had
been no thunder before, and very little during the autumn of 1793, whilft it raged
with fuch violence, and that the weather at
that time was exceffively hot and clofe. It
has been remarked all over North America,
that the weather had been much hotter in the
fummer and autumn of the two laft years,
and that there had been very little thunder
during all that time, in comparifon with former years; neither had there been any of the
ufual violent gales of wind upon the coaft
for the three preceding autumns.   In the

autumns of 1794 and 1795, this fever prevailed in Charles Town, Norfolk, and New
York; it broke out in the latter on the
arrival of great numbers from Ireland, and
in the two former, on the arrival of crowds
of emigrants from St. Domingo and the
other iſlands.   According to Dr. Lining's
account of this fever in Charles Town,
South Carolina, communicated in the Eſſays
Phyſical and Literary, Vol. II. it appears
to have broke out there in the years 1732,
1739, 1745, and 1748; he thinks it was
always imported from the Weſt Indies, but
gives no proof, or even reaſon, in ſupport
of this opinion, which does not ſeem to be
well founded.

5thly. This fever has not prevailed much
in theſe Windward Caribbee Iſlands for
many years paſt.   At Fort Royal, in Martinique, where there is a great prevalence
of mephitic effluvia, ariſing from the
marſhy ground at the back of the town, it
generally broke out in the ſummer or autumnal ſeaſon, on the arrival of troops from
France, or of a number of ſeamen, who never

ver had been in the West Indies before;
and the same thing happened at Point à
Petre, in Grand Terre, Guadaloupe, almost
annually, and from the same cause; but it
was never looked upon as an infectious
disease, nor did it ever spread among the
natives of the towns, or among those who
were seasoned to the climate, nor was it
ever carried from thence to the other
islands. In this island but few cases have occurred for these last twenty years, and these
have chiefly been at Prince Rupert's Head,
where, from the stagnated water in a large
morass near the town and fort, the marsh
miasma prevails in a high degree. Since
the swampy places which were in the town
of Roseau have been filled up, this fever
has been seldom observed; but previous to
the year 1792, we had generally violent
thunder storms, heavy rains, or severe gales
of wind, during the autumnal season.

M. Disportes, in his Histoire des Mala-
dies de St. Domingue, during the fourteen
years that he kept a journal of the diseases at
Cap François and Fort Dauphin, found that

E 3   this

this fever broke out conftantly in thefe towns upon the arrival of new-comers from France, and among thefe, only fuch as had not been formerly in that climate; and at the time it raged, which was chiefly during the autumn, the old feafoned inhabitants were only attacked with bilious remittents, and, what he terms, the lymphatic fever, which feems to have been more of the typhus kind, than of the bilious, but very different from the yellow fever. Dyfentery alfo prevailed among the feafoned inhabitants at the fame time. In and about thefe towns, during thefe fourteen years, viz. from the year 1732 to 1746, there were a great many inlets of the fea, where the water continued long in a ftagnated ftate, which in fo hot a place produced very offenfive exhalations; to thefe he attributes this fever, and the bilious and other difeafes that prevailed at the fame time. He mentions little in regard to the general ftate of the weather, or even as to gales of wind, or thunder and rain, and having no thermometer, he could give no accurate account of the degrees of heat.

6thly.

6thly. I have obferved, for many years
paft in this ifland, that when we had much
thunder and very heavy rains in the months
of June and July, we always efcaped a hurricane, or a fevere gale of wind. On the
contrary, if we had fine weather in thefe
months, we had either a hurricane, or a very
fickly feafon after. If that fevere fcourge
of the inhabitants of the Weft Indies took
place, by which the whole country was
laid wafte, and defolation was every where
to be feen, the inhabitants had better
health, than is ufual at that time of the
year, to compenfate them for their great
loffes and calamities. This was obferved
in all the iflands that fuffered by the fevere
hurricane of 1780. It was verified here; although we had only, what is called, the tail
of it. And in the year 1787, after two very
violent hurricanes in one week in this ifland,
the inhabitants were extremely healthy;
but it was health dearly purchafed.

7th. In the months of June, July, and
Auguft 1794, we had fome flight thun-
der ftorms, and this town was not fo un-
E 4   healthy

healthy afterwards; although many had this fever, and some died of it. In the same months in 1795, the thunder was more severe; we had bilious complaints and intermittent fevers all over the island, but this fever almost disappeared; and only a few cases occurred afterwards. I have had no information in regard to the state of the weather either in Jamaica or St. Domingo, during the three last years, that this fever has proved so destructive to our countrymen there.

By the excessive and long continued heat of the sun, the state of the atmosphere appears to be so much vitiated in all warm climates, that if some agent or means were not employed from time to time by nature to rectify it, these countries would become unfit for the residence of human beings.

Thunder, heavy rains, and violent gales of wind seem to be the agents for this purpose; which are the causes of restoring that due mixture of parts to the atmosphere, so indispensably necessary for the support of health.

A strong

A ftrong gale of wind, which is the moft
powerful inftrument made ufe of for ef-
fecting this purpofe in all climates, and
which, from its periodical or frequent returns in the warm feafon, is called in the
Eaft Indies and about the coaft of Africa,
tornado; in the Mediterranean fea, levan-
ter; on the coaft of North America, north-
wefter; and in the Windward and Leeward
Weft India Iflands, hurricane. Thefe winds
produce but too often the moft dreadful
effects both by fea and land, but they feem
to be directed by Providence for the good
of the whole, at the expence of the few.
The other agents anfwer likewife the purpofe of purifying the air, although in a
much lefs degree. The want of thefe cor-
rectives, as they may be termed, for impure air, left it in a ftate truly obnoxious
to general health, which I think was,
moft probably, the remote caufe of this
fever.

It was remarked, after the arrival of fuch
multitudes of people at Rofeau, at the time
when this fever had begun to rage with violence,

lence, that the air had a flat kind of fmell, and
that people foon became faintifh in it, on ufing
even very moderate exercife. This induced
me to make trial of the air, by Mr. Scheele's
fimple apparatus, not having a proper eudiometer. The purity of the air is perhaps afcertained more accurately in this
way, than it can be by the nitrous gas,
which depends fo much upon a variety of
circumftances in the feparation of it from
the acid of nitre. I filled, at different times,
gallipots with liver of fulphur, and alfo
with iron filings and flower of fulphur well
mixed and moiftened, and put thefe upon a
ftand under a glafs veffel, which was placed
on a ftool in a pail of water. The glafs veffel
was marked and divided on the outfide, and
allowance being made for the fpace that
the gallipot occupied, the water rofe only
one-fifth in the glafs veffel, after ftanding
twenty-four hours. When the difeafe abated, it rofe near one-fourth; and upon many
trials afterwards, when the place became
more healthy, the water never rofe above
one-fourth, which makes about twenty-
five

five parts of vital air that was taken up, but perhaps it was not entirely abforbed.

The air in the mountains of this ifland is very pure, and remarkably falubrious. I afcertained the heights very accurately of the places in the vicinity of the town, where the inhabitants were never attacked with any fever, but of the catarrhal or inflammatory kind, and where the people live to a great age; and to which, when the emigrants had fled, they always avoided an attack of fever, or foon recovered if in a convalefcent ftate: The elevations are as follow:

Feet high above the
level of the fea.

No.	Place	Feet	Description
1.	Bruce's Hill - - -	360	{ Pleafant and healthy, but not fo much fo as Daxon's Hill.
2.	The outer Cabritt, at Prince Rupert's Head, is - - -	600	{ More healthy than the inner Cabritt, and pleafant.
3.	Daxon's Hill - - -	1010	Very healthy.
4.	One Tree Hill, and the environs about the fame height - -	1300	{ Remarkably healthy.
5.	Mount Pleafant Eft -	1360	Ditto.
6.	Petit's Houfe, called Teneriff - -	2050	{ Cold and rather damp, and not fo healthy as the other places.

The places alluded to above.

Although

Although ſituations only from 400 to 600 feet above the level of the ſea are healthy and pleaſant. yet it appears from the foregoing experiments, that the air is purer and more healthy from the height of 1400 to 1500 feet, than it is when much below or above that height; in the latter caſe it becomes damp and raw, and by experience I find the inhabitants are not ſo healthy in ſuch high ſituations. I could not aſcertain the proportion of vital air in the atmoſphere at theſe heights, for want of a proper eudiometer; Mr. Scheele's apparatus having been found quite inconvenient for that purpoſe; but this I will endeavour to have tried exactly, on ſome future occaſion. If the troops on their arrival in the Weſt Indies could be quartered in ſuch high ſituations for a little time, till they got accuſtomed to the heat of the climate by degrees, ſo many of them would not be loſt. Where this is impracticable, they ſhould if poſſible be landed in theſe iſlands in the month of December or January, which are the cooleſt times of the year.

　　　　　　　　　　Theory.

Theory. This derangement of the component parts of the atmofphere, was probably effected by the ftrong light and intenfe heat of the * fun having difengaged, or formed fome combination with its vital part, or a certain portion of it, which being fo united and rarified, would rife far above that ftratum of air, in which we, in lower fituations, breathe, leaving the mephitic or heavier part near to the furface of the earth. The lofs of a fmall portion of vital air, would render this lower ftratum very unfit for refpiration, and of courfe very unwholefome to live in.—The atmofphere of this town became probably vitiated in this manner by degrees, and therefore did not affect the health of the inhabitants either fuddenly, or.very confiderably. The common remittent fever, dyfentery, and other bilious complaints, had, however, begun to fhow themfelves, previous to the appearance of the yellow fever.

* M. de Fourcroy's Preliminary Difcourfe, in his Elements of Natural Hiftory and Chemiftry.

The

The air already thus deranged, was, by the
fudden arrival of a number of perfons greatly
exhaufted, and unprovided with changes of
cloathing, and alfo crowded together in an
extraordinary manner, fo contaminated with
mephitic exhalations, and exalted to fuch a
pitch of malignancy, that all who had been
accuftomed to breathe a purer air, viz. the
Europeans, Americans, thofe from high fituations in the mountains, as well as the
emigrants, who, as mentioned before, were
predifpofed by a multiplicity of caufes,
would all be readily and greatly affected by
it. If the conftitution is able to refift the
firft attacks of the common bilious remittent fever, occafioned by refiding in the
neighbourhood of marfhy places, experience has fhown us that by habit the hane-
ful influence of thefe mephitic vapours will
be entirely overcome, and that fuch perfons
having efcaped fome attacks of this kind, may
continue to live in fuch an atmofphere, and
enjoy as good health, as people in general
do, in Weft India towns. But the animal
œconomy is not only influenced by habit in
all its parts, but it has alfo a power of con-
formity

formity to almoſt any change, either of increaſe or decreaſe of nouriſhment, or of la-
bour, as well as of reſt, confinement, want
of ſleep, &c. &c. as it has alſo of breathing
a foul unwholeſome air with little apparent
injury to health, provided any or all of theſe
variations or ſtates of life, are brought about
gradually. The direction of our ideas, and
the powers of thinking and acting, are in
all caſes influenced by cuſtom. For theſe
reaſons, probably, new-comers are ſpeedily
attacked with this fever after their arrival,
even in places where it does not prevail,
and this gives it ſo much the appearance of
an infectious diſeaſe, where it has already
broke out.

A deranged ſtate of the atmoſphere, as
mentioned before, ſeemed to me to be the
firſt cauſe that excited this mortal diſeaſe in
our iſland ; and as it prevailed in the different towns of the other iſlands, the more
they were crowded with ſtrangers, I am inclined to believe, that it proceeded from the
ſame cauſe in them all, aided, and perhaps
put in action, by the great concourſe of
people

people in towns expoſed to ſo much heat. New-comers from Europe, in high health, were ſooneſt affected by this impure air, others, who had reſided ſome time in un-wholeſome places in America, and in the French iſlands, reſiſted its baleful influence much longer; and perhaps, by the extra-ordinary or immoderate accumulation of it, in ſome Weſt India and American towns, even the old inhabitants were ſometimes affected with this fever. In this way, many fevers of the typhus kind may become more or leſs epidemic, which are not in themſelves contagious, as is always the caſe in the jail and ſhip fevers. I believe the air did never arrive at that contagious de-gree of accumulated impurity in this iſland: For when patients labouring under this fe-ver, were removed to high ſituations for the ſake of breathing a cooler and purer air, and who, notwithſtanding, fell victims to it, the people about them were never infected, nor did the diſeaſe ever prevail afterwards in ſuch places.——And I have been aſſured that this was exactly the caſe in America. There appears to have been ſuch an exten-

live

five and very peculiar deranged state of the
atmosphere in the towns in these islands,
and in North America, that it is more proba-
ble, this disease was produced by this general
cause, breaking out nearly at the same time
in different places, than that it originated
only in one or two towns, and was carried
from thence by infection to others, by either
persons or goods, as has been supposed.
The regular return, and continuance, of
this fever in the months of July, August,
and September, every year, more or less,
since its first appearance in these islands,
and in the towns in America, seems to me
to argue strongly in favour of this opinion.
From these facts and observations I am of
opinion, that in all hot climates, where a
great depravity of the atmosphere is produced by the causes already mentioned, and
where its natural purifiers are wanting, this
fever will break out in such places, on the
arrival of a great number of strangers, more
especially if they come from a cold country.
If such impure air is allowed to be the remote cause of this fever, as appears from
what has been said; the air in respiration, in

F   this

this case, not having a sufficient quantity of oxygene, may occasion a deranged state of the fluids, which I conceive to be the immediate stimulus or excitement, or what may be termed the proximate cause of this fever. And if the biliary secretion be intended for the discharge of the degenerated lymph and crassamentum of the blood, as Dr. Maclurg thinks, in his dissertation on the bile; the great redundancy and degeneracy of the bile in this fever may be easily accounted for on that principle. This derangement may be the cause of an increased determination of the fluids to the liver, and as the morbid animal process gains ground, which it does every hour, if not opposed by powerful remedies, the liver becomes more and more distended with blood, and the biliary secretion is increased and hurried on in such a rapid manner through the extremities of the pori biliari, that it resembles grounds of coffee rather than bile, which, upon a narrow inspection with a magnifying glass, seemed to be black dissolved blood, floating in lymph or mucus. When the blood, dissolved by this morbid
                                        process,

procefs, meets with any obftruction, it
gufhes from the nofe and mouth in almoft
a colourlefs ftate, and in fuch prodigious
quantities, that the patient foon finks into a
ftate of total diffolution.

Query. Is it poffible to difcover a method to purify the atmofphere of a town,
or to deprive it of the fuperabundant quantity of mephitic gas, fo deftructive to animal
life ?

Fire has been formerly employed as a
purifier of the air, wherever great malignancy of it was fufpected; but fince the
difcoveries of the late Monf. Lavoifier and
others, fhewing that combuftion deprives
it of a portion of the vital part fo effential
to life, fome doubts may be entertained
in regard to the propriety of ufing great
fires on fuch occafions. But it may ftill
be a queftion, whether the good effects of
fire, efpecially in fhips and clofe chambers,
may not be accounted for from the rarefac-
tion and confequent influx of frefh air which
it occafions ?

F 2   Burning

Burning of brimstone and other combustible substances in the holds of ships, and also in prisons and hospitals where bad air prevailed, has been found useful in purifying it. Might not a large fire of wood placed twice a day at the leeward side of hospitals, where the sick of this fever are, be of some service in purifying the air? Leaves of vegetables wetted and placed in the sun s rays in the windows and doors on the windward side of hospitals or houses where the sick are placed, in the West Indies, as mentioned before, may contribute in a small degree also to purify the air. Perhaps the explosion of gunpowder in some convenient parts of the towns in the West Indies and America where this fever prevails, two or three times a day, would be useful in a general way ; or, what is better, the deflagration of nitre, or small quantities of moist gunpowder, might be useful to purify hospitals in the inside, or to the leeward of them, in houses and in private practice. This might be tried at a small expence in the West India islands, where cannon powder is so soon damaged in the different gar-

rifons

rifons by the exceffive humidity of the air, at fome feafons of the year.

But all artificial means yet difcovered can avail but little, and even the frequent thunder ftorms that we have had for thefe two years paft, which, although of infinite ufe in moderating the difeafe, feem to be too weak agents to reftore the atmofphere to its wonted falubrity. A hurricane, that terrible fcourge of the Weft India planter, appears to be the only agent now fufficiently powerful to effect that purpofe. And a violent gale of wind (called north wefter), together with fevere thunder ftorms, on the fouthern part of North America, are equally neceffary to diffipate the impure air in their towns, and thereby remove from them, for a term of years, this dreadful difeafe.

OF

OF THE

BILIOUS REMITTENT
FEVER
OF THE *WEST INDIES.*

===

CHAPTER I.

SECTION I.

THIS Fever is the fame in all the Weft India iflands, and probably in all hot climates, differing only in the degree of violence, according to the greater or lefs prevalence of its remote caufe, which I conceive to be marfh effluvia.

The Symptoms.

IT begins with a chillinefs, giddinefs, and head-ach ; fenfe of great weaknefs, ficknefs at the ftomach, and pain of the back. There is a peculiar uneafy fenfation all over the

the furface of the body; the eyes look heavy, the countenance is pale and dejected, the ſkin dry, and the pulſe feeble and very quick. Great anxiety and reſtleſſneſs ſoon follow; and when the ſenſe of cold wears off, a violent vomiting of yellow or green bile comes on. The contents of the ſtomach are generally thrown up during the chilly fit, together with what the patient has drank, for the thirſt is then very great. The heat of the body is now increaſed; the pulſe becomes fuller, the face fluſhed, and a redneſs of the ſkin appears, particularly about the breaſt. The tongue is dry and white, and in grown people the pulſe is generally from 90 to 100 ſtrokes in a minute. The patient becomes extremely reſtleſs, the vomiting is inceſſant, and ſometimes a delirium comes on. In this ſtate the ſick remain from 8 to 12 hours, about which time a ſlight moiſture appears, firſt on the face and breaſt, and afterwards by degrees all over the body. When the ſweat was general, and continued for an hour or two, and the vomiting ceaſed, a remiſſion of fever followed. But more frequently the

F 4   ſweating

ſweating was partial, and did not continue long; the pungent heat on the ſkin remained, the vomiting was renewed, and the paroxyſm prolonged for 8 or 12 hours more. The urine is always high coloured from the very firſt ſymptom of the diſeaſe, and continues ſo throughout. The firſt paroxyſm generally begins in the evening, or about eleven o'clock A M. The patient is languid and confuſed after the firſt fit, his ſkin ſoon becomes dry, the heat continues to be greater than natural, he is not quite free from head-ach, and on ſitting up or walking about, he feels a dizzineſs in it. This remiſſion generally continued for 8 or 12 hours, when another paroxyſm came on, ſometimes with a ſenſe of coldneſs, but more frequently with a great ſenſe of heat all over the body; the head-ach increaſed, and the vomiting ſoon became more violent than it was in the firſt fit. All the ſymptoms were now much more violent, and the paroxyſm generally continued 18 or 24 hours, when a ſweat came on; which, if profuſe, a remiſſion followed. When the patient had not taken any medicine, this remiſſion

miffion was of fhort duration, feldom con-
tinuing more than 4 or 6 hours. In the
third fit there was feldom any rigor, the
exacerbation came on with violent vomiting, increafed head-ach and heat, and all the
febrile fymptoms were much higher; the
tongue became very dry and foul, the thirft
intolerable, and the eyes more inflamed;
which fymptom, however, difappeared during the remiffion. The delirium and anxiety were increafed, and the enfuing remiffion was very imperfect, running into a
fourth exacerbation or paroxyfm in a few
hours, which often proved fatal on the fifth
day, if no medicine or bark had been given
from the beginning, or if the patient had
been treated improperly, by bleeding, warm
baths, or large dofes of emetic tartar. The
patient in this cafe either became quite delirious, or fell into a comatofe ftate. At
the height of this paroxyfm the heat is
greatly increafed, and fo pungent, that a
difagreeable fenfation remains upon the ends
of the fingers after feeling the patient's
pulfe and fkin. The pulfe now beats 120
times in a minute; and towards the clofe of
the

the scene, I have counted it at 130 or 140. The breathing is now very laborious; and there is generally a subsultus tendinum, trembling of the hands, feeling the bed cloaths, catching at something in the air, staring, talking and muttering, till the patient is snatched off suddenly by a sort of convulsion; or they sometimes remained in an insensible state for many hours, breathing with great difficulty till they expired. Coldness of the extremities, and cold sweats, are always symptoms of great danger, and seldom fail to appear in the last stage of this disease. I have never observed petechiæ; but some hours before death the sick had a cadaverous smell, the face and extremities put on a livid appearance, and the stools were very offensive. I have never met with any patients in this fever who had a bleeding at the nose, and though hiccup is very common, yet it is not always a mortal symptom, as it is in the yellow fever. Musqueto bites, and prickly heat, generally disappear on the first attack. A suppression of urine does not come on, nor is it ever of a yellow colour, as in the yellow fever, except in such as have the

jaundice

jaundice as a concomitant fymptom. On the contrary, it is remarkably high colour-ed, refembling porter, both during the re-miffions and in the paroxyfms. When the fever came on without any rigor or chilly fit, the greater was the danger; the remiffions being more imperfect. The contrary of which happened in the yellow-fever. When there was much rain in the months of May and June, and dry fultry weather prevailed in the following months of July and Auguft, this fever raged much among the troops and ftrangers, and fometimes proved fatal when not attended to at the beginning, or when improperly treated. In general, how-ever, it was not fo very violent or rapid in its progrefs as defcribed above; it refembled a double tertian intermittent, with this differ-ence, that the paroxyfms were much longer and more violent, and the intermiffions were never fo perfect, or fo clearly mark-ed. When the remiffions and paroxyfms fucceeded one another fo rapidly that there was little time to adminifter the bark, a dofe or two of James's or the antimonial powder, and a blifter between the fhoulders,

generally

generally brought about an intermiſſion or
a good remiſſion, and then the bark was
adminiſtered as quickly as poſſible, and generally with ſuccefs.   In young children this
fever ſometimes came on with a convulſion
fit, or they had one when the hot fit was at
its height; which being frequently ſup-
poſed to proceed from worms, and being
treated for ſuch, precious time was loſt, and
the diſeaſe thereby often proved fatal.   A
fever proceeding from worms in the Weſt
Indies I never found to be very violent, or
ever preceded by a cold fit, nor were there
any remiſſions or exacerbations. This ought
to be ſtrictly attended to; as many children
have been loſt from this miſtake.   The
voiding of worms is no certain indication
that the diſeaſe proceeds from them, although it is a very difficult matter to per-
ſuade the parents or nurſes that it does
not.   The more violent and diſtinct the
paroxyſms, the greater certainty there is
that it is really of the remittent kind. Some
grown people had a ſenſe of torpor, or
numbneſs in their extremities upon the firſt
attack of this fever, and others had a temporary privation of ſight, which occaſioned
great

great alarm; but thefe fymptoms were not followed by fatal confequences, probably owing to the great care, and extraordinary attention that was paid to thofe who were attacked in this feemingly dangerous way.

I have feen many inftances of a yellow-nefs of the eyes coming on, and fpreading all over the body about the fifth day, which was at firft a very alarming fymptom; but by experience it was found not to be a dangerous one. It ought to be obferved, however, that in thefe cafes, the paroxyfms and remiffions of fever were clearly and diftinct-ly marked; and alfo, that in thofe who died of it, the black-vomit never appeared, as it did conftantly and uniformly in all cafes of the yellow-fever which proved fatal. The yellownefs coming on in a fever, with evident remiffions and paroxyfms, may be therefore looked upon as only an accidental jaundice, and unconnected with it in any other way; which is far from being the cafe in the yellow-fever.

Although

Although some medical gentlemen have
supposed the yellow-fever to be contagious,
as I observed in my history of it; few, if any,
I believe, will contend for this fever being
so.   In these islands, no practitioner of my
acquaintance entertains any such opinion;
and I am fully convinced, from long experience, that it is not infectious. The constant
supply of fresh air by the trade-winds, and
sea and land breezes, probably render dif-
eases very seldom contagious in this climate.
The effluvia from rich low lands after much
rain, have nearly the same effects upon the
human constitution in producing this fever,
as the marsh miasmata, or the vapours from
stagnated water about the mouths of rivers
or inlets of the sea have, only differing in
degree. These bring on intermittents more
or less violent, while the strong marsh effluvia produce this fever.   Strangers are
more liable to the deleterious influence of
these mephitic vapours than the natives are,
or those who have been seasoned to such climates, as was observed of the yellow-fever;
but there seems something different in the
general

general ſtate of the atmoſphere, as mentioned before, which renders it leſs dangerous. While this fever attacked ſtrangers in
July and the autumnal months, the natives
and ſeaſoned inhabitants were ſometimes
attacked with intermittents.

The uniform and regular diſpoſition to
remit, eaſily and readily diſtinguiſhes this
from the yellow-fever. Neither the redneſs of the eyes, nor the fluſhing of the
face, are ſo remarkable, and they always
diſappear during the remiſſions. The reſpi-
ration is laborious during the paroxyſm,
and the pulſe always quick and hard, which
is never the caſe in the yellow-fever. A
conſtant vomiting of bile accompanies every
paroxyſm of this fever from the very firſt
attack, which does not happen ſo early in
the other. This is an invariable ſymptom
throughout the diſeaſe. And farther, a remiſſion or evident abatement of the febrile
ſymptoms, takes place always in the courſe
of twelve hours after the firſt attack, and
the paroxyſm is renewed ſome hours after,
which is never the caſe in the yellow-
                                        fever,

fever, as I have fhewn in the firft part of this work.

SECTION II.

Of the Cure of the Remittent Fever.

As there is generally a want of appetite, always a ficknefs of the ftomach, head-ach, an uneafy feeling all over the body, or fome indifpofition for a day or two before the firft attack ; five or fix grains of calomel at this period, and a brifk purgative given eight hours after, will often entirely prevent the fever, or abate its violence confiderably if it comes on, fo that the conftitution will not be injured by it; efpecially if fix or eight dofes of bark are taken daily for three or four days after the purgative. When called during the firft paroxyfm, if the retching and vomiting were violent, a few cupsful of camomile tea were given to cleanfe the ftomach ; and foon after, a purging draught, confifting of from one to

two

two scruples of jalap in cinnamon or mint
water. If this did not remain long enough
on the stomach to have the desired effect,
a clyster was ordered, and ten grains of
calomel and half a dram of jalap made up
into ten pills, four of which were given at
first, and two every half hour afterwards
till they operated. These were seldom vomited up, and were found to be the most
efficacious purge of any that was tried.
The neutral salts were so often vomited up,
that I have laid them aside altogether for
some years past, and used the draught or pills,
which has answered the purpose much better. Six or eight stools procured by these
means relieved the head-ach and vomiting,
a sweat generally followed, and with it a
remission of all the febrile symptoms. The
use of the Peruvian bark was begun as early
as possible, in substance, if the stomach
would bear it, or in small doses of the
powder in two ounces of a strong decoction
or infusion of it every hour or hour and a half
during the remission. It was sometimes
necessary to give an anodyne draught after
the purgative, to quiet the stomach previ-

G ous

ous to giving the bark. At other times a cup of fago or panada with wine, anfwered the purpofe of fettling the ftomach. The pale bark in fubftance was preferred to the red, although the latter made the ftrongeft decoction or infufion, which was given when the powder would not fit on the ftomach. If an ounce of bark in fubftance, or half that quantity in a pint of the ftrong decoction or infufion, was retained on the ftomach during the firft remiffion, the fecond paroxyfm would not be very fevere, and the fame quantity given in the fecond remiffion, would generally prevent a third fit. Purgatives ought conftantly to be employed during or towards the decline of the paroxyfm, in order not to lofe time in giving the bark, when the remiffion takes place. It is however worthy of obfervation, that it requires a very large dofe of any purgative to have a proper effect during the hot fit of the fever; and on that account the purgatives were generally poftponed till the violence of the paroxyfm was over. When the patient was not vifited till the firft remiffion, and no medicine had been

I

given,

given, a purging clyfter was ordered; and a
dofe of bark made purgative by the addition of ten or fifteen grains of jalap was
given immediately, and the bark in fubftance or otherwife, was adminiftered as often as the ftomach could bear it afterwards.
If not called to the fick till the fecond paroxyfm, a purgative was ordered; or if he
had been purged during the remiffion,
which generally happened, five * grains of
James's powder or eight grains of the pulv.
antimonialis were given to an adult, and
repeated every two or three hours, till
fome fenfible effect was produced by it. A
grain or grain and a half of pure opium was
frequently given to fettle the ftomach after
the antimonial, and to prepare it to retain
the bark, which was always exhibited as
foon as poffible.

When the head ach was very violent in this
paroxyfm, and more efpecially if the patient

* I am inclined to think from repeated trials, that
one-third part more is required of the p. antimonialis
Londinenfis, than of the James's powder, to produce the
fame effect on the fame perfon.

was delirious, a large blister was applied to the neck, which seldom failed to remove both. If the vomiting became more severe about the end of this, or the beginning of the third paroxysm, and could not be restrained by saline draughts in the act of effervescence, or by a grain or two of solid opium, a blister was applied over the epigastric region, which seldom failed to put a stop to it in a few hours. Mustard was applied over the pit of the stomach, when blistering on that part was not thought safe or proper, and it often had a very good effect. The bark was mixed up in different vehicles, according to the taste or whim of the sick, as in wine, wine and water, porter, toast and water, &c.; but in general cold coffee with a little sugar, covered the taste of it better than any other liquid, and made it sit more easily on the stomach. The taste of it is also very well covered by milk, and in this way it was commonly given to delicate people and to children. When the bark purged, five drops of laudanum were added to each dose, or fifteen drops to the first dose, which never failed

to

to prevent its running off that way. If on the contrary it occasioned costiveness, some calcined magnesia was rubbed with the bark, or five grains of jalap added to a dose or two every day, which kept the bowels sufficiently open. The same quantity of jalap seemed to purge more when joined to the bark, than when given alone. The infusion of bark was made with boiling water, when wanted quickly, and at other times it was made in cold water, in lime water, or with magnesia in water.

When the stomach rejected the bark in every form, which sometimes happened, it was given in clysters, either in a strong decoction cold, with some of the powder, or the powder mixed up in thin starch jelly. In the former case two drams of the powder with the decoction, and in the latter half an ounce of the powder, were thrown up every two hours, thirty or forty drops of laudanum having been previously added to the first clyster, to prevent their being speedily discharged. By this method many were saved, who would have died, if no

G 3

attempt

attempt had been made to employ the
bark, when the ftomach had conftantly rejected it after repeated trials. The bark
was applied externally all over the abdomen
of children as well as given in clyfters, when
they could not keep it on their ftomachs;
and they generally paffed a number of worms
by the purgative of jalap and calomel given
previous to the bark. When no bark had
been given during the third remiffion, the
fucceeding paroxyfm was very violent, and
a delirium or coma enfued, in which cafe a
blifter was applied to the head, and finapifms
to the feet and hands, The great debility
at this period very often prevented our attempting to ufe the James's or antimonial
powder, although it was fometimes adminiftered with fuccefs in cafes that were
looked upon as defperate. But in general, as
much bark, wine, and nourifhment at intervals, was given as the ftomach would
bear. A hiccup was a common fymptom
at this period, and it was always very diftreffing to the patient, and in fome inftances continued to the laft moment of
his exiftence. It was often relieved by
laudanum,

laudanum, and fometimes by mufk. Camphor was always hurtful by irritating the ftomach, and increafing that dreadful fymptom an inceffant vomiting.

After the patient had been purged, and dangerous or alarming fymptoms appeared, the bark was given at all times when the ftomach would bear it, and it was applied in every way, without any regard to remiffions or exacerbations of fever. Nourifhment and wine was given between each dofe of bark, or as often as poffible, and frefh air admitted into the chambers of the fick by every means. When a paroxyfm was attended with only a flight delirium, but with great reftleffnefs and anxiety, thirty or forty drops of laudanum gave great relief, and often brought about a fweat and remiffion of fever.

I have never bled any perfon in this fever, and although I have heard of venefection being employed with fuccefs on fome young robuft men, when attacked foon after their arrival from Europe, yet I am of opinion that

G 4   it

it is fo hazardous an operation that it ought hardly ever to be attempted. I have been confirmed in this opinion from having feen thofe to whom I have been called, after they had been bled, almoft always in fuch a ftate of debility, that no cordials or any means whatever were fufficiently powerful to prevent their finking entirely in the fucceeding paroxyfm. Emetic tartar increafes the irratibility of the ftomach, and ought never to be ufed in any ftage of this difeafe. I have known many fall victims to the imprudent, or rafh application as it will perhaps be called, of this medicine; but as we have fafer remedies at hand, it is better to lay afide the ufe of it entirely in this fever. When the ftomack is foul, and the bile that is thrown up is very thick and ropy, I have ordered an infufion of ipecacuanha with a view to cleanfe it, which this fimple medicine always effected without increafing its irritability.

In general, very few died of this fever, who were treated in the manner here recommended; and I think I can aver with truth, that I have not loft more than one

patient

patient out of fifty, when I have been called to their afliftance during the firft or fecond paroxyfm, and even very few after the third. Much, however, depends on the early and liberal adminiftration of he bark. Though I have never been able to obferve any thing like critical days in this fever, yet I have never known any perfon die of it after the eighth day.

If the bark was not continued daily for a week or ten days after the fever was ftopt, an intermittent of the double tertian or quartan type came on, which was very difficult to be removed, rendered the patient very weak and his convalefcence very long. It is abfolutely neceffary to enforce the ufe of the bark for fome time after, and to keep the bowels open until the ftrength is thoroughly reftored. Camomile or fnake-root tea, to which fometimes elixir of vitriol was added, every morning early, and at eleven o'clock, contributed much to reftore the appetite. Riding on horfeback every morning early, and removing to a high fituation in the country when it could be done conveniently, was always recommended.

If

If, as before mentioned, the indifpofition previous to an attack of this fever be attended to, and five or fix grains of James's powder, or fix or eight grains of calomel to a robuft perfon be given before the fever is formed, and a purgative next day, an attack may generally be prevented. Or if the fkin is very dry, and there is already fome fever, a good dofe of the antimonial or James's powder will anfwer the purpofe better, and by purging and fweating, prepare the patient for the ufe of the bark, which ought never to be omitted.

CHAP-

CHAPTER II.

SECTION I.

Of Intermittent Fevers.

I HAVE not met with a regular quotidian fever in this ifland ; the fit generally came on in the morning of one day, and in the afternoon of the fucceeding, and when particular attention was paid to the fymptoms, the firft paroxyfm was found to be more violent than the fecond, and the fever feemed to partake much of the double tertian type.

In the moft regular tertian type of this fever, there is generally fome anxiety and uneafinefs, or a flight febrile attack, about eleven o'clock in the forenoon, or in the evening of the day of the intermiffion, which is not often attended to, but conftitutes alfo in fome degree a double tertian type. In what is called the tertian ague, anticipations

of

of the paroxyſms are very common, which if not prevented by bark will run into one another, and form a real double tertian of a more or leſs dangerous tendency, according to the duration of the intermiſſions. From what I have obſerved of intermittents in this and ſome of the other Weſt India iſlands, I am inclined to think that the double tertian and the quartan types are the only real diſtinctions amongſt them. From my own experience I am alſo of opinion, that the remittent fever follows the ſame periods in regard to remiſſions, and paroxyſms or exacerbations, as the double tertian intermittent does, differing only from it in degree of violence.

The quartan type, in general, is very diſtinctly marked, its paroxyſms returning very nearly every ſeventy-two hours. The cold fit of an ague does not continue ſo long here as it generally does in cold climates, ſeldom exceeding half an hour ; but the longer it continues, the more complete and durable the ſucceeding intermiſſion always

ways is, and the lefs danger is to be appre-
hended.

Intermittents, when negle&ed or treated
improperly, bring on fixed affe&ions of the
liver, fuch as fenfible hardnefs and enlarge-
ment, and in fome cafes the fpleen is alfo
enlarged and hard. Thefe obftru&ions are
generally followed by dropfy, particularly
after the quartan.

Although purging is not a neceffary preparative to the ufe of the bark, a dofe of jalap
was generally given ; or if the patient had
vomited much bile during the former fit, a
calomel pill was ordered, and a purge of jalap
next morning. But in urgent cafes, where the
intermiffions were fhort, a fcruple of jalap
was ordered with the firft dofe of bark, and
the bark was given every hour or hour and
a half in dram dofes, during the intermiffion. When the tongue was very foul, and
a quantity of thick bile had been thrown
up in the former paroxyfm, half a dram of
ipecacuanha in powder, or an infufion of
two drams of the root in a tea-cup full of
boiling

boiling water, was ordered to be given on
the appearance of the firſt ſymptoms of the
cold fit, which not only cleanſed the ſtomach, but alſo ſhortened the paroxyſm, and
in ſome inſtances entirely removed the diſeaſe. A grain and a half or two grains of tartar emetic given to robuſt people, on the firſt
approach of the cold fit, produced frequently the ſame good effect. When the type
of the ague was aſcertained, I did not begin
the bark till eight or ten hours before the
ſevere fit of a double tertian, or twelve
hours before the fit of a quartan, giving a
dram in ſubſtance every hour or hour and a
half till the time the fit was expected, and
generally ſome doſes afterwards, as the bark
frequently retarded the paroxyſm and made
it leſs violent, when it had not ſufficient
powers to prevent it entirely. Thirty or
forty drops of laudanum given to a grown
perſon in the hot fit, had a good effect in
bringing on a ſweat ſpeedily, ſhortening the
fit, and ſettling the ſtomach, ſo as to enable
it to retain the bark better the next intermiſſion. The pale bark has been preferred
of late to the red, the latter having been
                                    found

found often to ruffle the ftomach and occa-
fion great uneafinefs in it. I have found
by experience, that an ounce of bark given
in the courfe of the eight or ten hours pre-
ceeding the paroxyfm of an intermittent, had
more effect in ftopping it, than double that
quantity had when taken at a confiderable
diftance of time before the cold fit. From
this fact well eftablifhed, I have been able
to cure intermittents with one half the
quantity of bark or lefs, than has been
ufually employed for that purpofe. Three
or four dofes taken on the fever days only,
a few hours previous to the time the fit was
expected, was fufficient in general to prevent
it; but to fecure the patient againft a relapfe, the bark ought to be continued in
this way for at leaft ten days or a fortnight
after the fit has been ftopped. If no more
bark is taken than what is barely fufficient
to ftop a paroxyfm, which, from the aver-
fion people in general have to this remedy,
is too often the cafe, a relapfe or return of
fever will take place the eighth day in the
double tertian, or what is commonly termed
the quotidian ague; and in the imperfect
double

double tertian, or tertian type, as it is called, the relapſe will happen on the fourteenth or fifteenth day, and in the quartan on the twenty-firſt or twenty-ſecond, making in each' type, nearly ſeven periodical revoſutions of the diſeaſe from the time the fit was ſtopped to the next attack. I have obſerved, when relapſes happened at this time, that on reckoning backwards the days and periods of the fever, it was found that the fit returned on the ſame day, and nearly at the ſame hour, that it would, if its courſe had not been interrupted from the commencement by the bark. Theſe relapſes will often happen independently of any irregularity of regimen, to which they are commonly imputed. I am inclined to aſcribe theſe periodical returns of intermittents, more to a certain habit contracted in the conſtitution, than to any influence of the moon over the body, as has been conceived by ſome phyſicians. But as great alterations in the weather generally take place about the changes of the moon in this climate, eſpecially in the autumn ; and as convaleſcents are more readily affected by ſuch viciſſitudes, I commonly ordered two

or

of three ounces of bark to be taken by thofe
recovering from an attack of fever, two or
three days before every full and new moon,
for fome months, which effectually prevented relapfes of this kind. It is neceffary to obferve here, that when intermittents
have been neglected or improperly treated
in the beginning, and are become fixed in
the habit, as it is generally termed, the
bark will not fucceed without the previous
ufe of mercury, as in fuch cafes obftructions
of the liver are brought on, efpecially in the
quartan type, as before obferved, which can
only be removed by a gentle courfe of mercury. I have known may inftances of quartans having been perfectly cured in this way.
When anafarca comes on after repeated attacks of a quartan, obftructions of the liver
are to be fufpected ; and if a hardnefs of the
liver or fpleen is difcovered on examination,
mercury fhould be adminiftered without lofs
of time, otherwife a confirmed dropfy will
foon follow, and the difeafe will prove fatal.
If the anafarca proceeds from debility, or
continues after the obftructions are removed, a change of climate becomes necefiary;

H fometimes

fometimes removing to the cool air of the mountains in this ifland, has anfwered the purpofe of reftoring the patient to health; but if circumftances will admit of a voyage to a colder climate, the reftoration of health will be more certain, and the opportunity of obtaining it ought not to be loft.

The bark of the cinchona caribæa, or cinchona brachycarpa, called country jefuits bark, both lately difcovered in this ifland, is alfo effectual in intermittent fevers. I have cured obftinate quartans with bark of the cinchona brachycarpa * in powder, and the tertian ague with the cold infufion of both of thefe barks; but when the brachycarpa is given to white people, it is neceffary to throw away the firft infufion, as it is extremely bitter, and feems to poffefs fomething of an emetic quality. The fecond infufion is not fo ftrong, but cures common intermittents in a few days. Upon eftates among the negroes, the firft infufion anfwers the pur-

* Some experiments have been made on this bark, by Mr. Brand, apothecary to the Queen, which will probably be publifhed.

8   pofe

pofe of a preparative to the ufe of the bark, as it commonly vomits and purges gently, and a quart of the fecond infufion given every day for two or three days after cures the fever. The cold fecond infufion is a good ftomachic, and may prove a very ufeful remedy for dyfpepfia. I prefer the bark of the cinchona brachycarpa, but it as well as the caribæa feems to be fomewhat deficient in the aftringent quality poffeffed by the cinchona officinalis ; I therefore fometimes added a little of the bark of the * prunus fpharofpermus, called bois tanne by the French, being a large tree, the bark of which is ufed for tanning leather, to the infufion, which I fuppofed contributed to render it a more powerful febrifuge.

The white arfenicated drops, prepared as directed in the London Medical Journal, fucceeded very well in a few cafes of inter-mittents, but it has not been brought into

---

* The bark of the prunus fpharofpermus is remarkably aftringent, probably more fo than the oak bark. It is ufed in decoction to check diarrhœa or licnteria.

general

general ufe yet in thefe iflands.   It bids fair
however to be a ufeful remedy among the
negroes, and robuft hardy people. The fafeft
method of ufing it in the Weft Indies,
where the nurfes are generally negro women, is to mix it with water, fo that a
table fpoonful of the mixture may contain
five drops, by which means miftakes will
be avoided.

CHAP.

CHAPTER III.

SECTION I.

Of the Typhus Fever.

FEW cafes of the real Nervous Fever have occurred in this or the other iflands, as I have been informed, for many years paft. When it has occured in this ifland, keeping the patient open in his bowels, bliftering the head repeatedly, giving a decoction of bark and fnake root, and fupporting the ftrength with nourifhment and wine, were the means employed for the cure; and in general with fuccefs. Two cafes occurred where the difeafe was protracted to the twentieth day, and both recovered. In fome of the other iflands, as I have been informed by medical gentlemen, it has been treated with great fuccefs, by throwing cold fea-water over the patients, three or four times a day, in the manner directed by Dr. William Wright, late of Edinburgh, now phyfician to the army in

H 3   the

the Weſt Indies, a ſituation he is well qua-
liſied for.

SECTION II.

PLEURISY, Piripneumony, and Catarrhal
Fevers, and Gaſtratis, &c. have not occurred
often in this iſland. When there are evident
ſymptoms of local inflammation, bleeding
largely and frequently is abſolutely necef-
ſary, eſpecially in the pleuriſy; and ſtrong
doſes of the antimonial or James's powder
and calomel were given afterwards, other-
wiſe the diſeaſe proved ſpeedily fatal.   Fomentations and bliſtering the ſide affected
muſt not be neglected; and cooling emo-
lient drinks, ſuch as barley-water with
ockra, to which ſome nitre is added, ſhould
be given frequently. The blood in this and
the hepatitis, which has occurred often in
this iſland*, had always a thick inflammatory
buff upon it. If bleeding is not uſed very

* See my paper on abſceſſes and diſeaſes of the liver
in the Weſt Indies in Decade 2d, Vol. IV. p. 317, of
Edinburgh Medical Commentaries.

early

early and plentifully in gaſtratis, a mortification of the bowels ſoon follows, and the
patient is carried off in the courſe of three
days illneſs.

A catarrhal fever, called a cold, ſeldom
requires bleeding; but a doſe or two of
P. antimonialis or James's powder is very
often neceſſary to remove it. Ten grains
of the former, or ſix of the latter, was the
common doſe given to grown people.

Bleeding in the acute hepatitis ſhould be
employed very early and largely, as well
as in the pleuriſy, to prevent an abſceſs
forming in the liver.

As the dyſentery generally prevails at the
ſame time that remittent and intermittent
fevers do, in the Weſt Indies, and probably
proceeds from the ſame cauſe, I ſhall next
give a ſhort account of the method of treatment that I have found moſt ſucceſsful in
that diſeaſe for many years paſt.

H 4   CHAP-

CHAPTER IV.

SECTION I.

Of the Dysentery.

THE accurate description that has been given of this disease by so many eminent authors, renders it unnecessary for me to enter upon the diagnosis; I shall therefore proceed to the method of cure.

I have never found occasion to use venesection. If the fever ran high, and the excruciating pain and griping in the bowels were not relieved by warm fomentations and emollient clysters, the semicupium was ordered, which never failed to alleviate them for a time, but it was seldom repeated, as it evidently weakened the patient: on which account, when the pain returned with violence, a blister was generally applied over the abdomen. While these applications were employed to palliate the disease, difeafe, an infufion of ipecacuanha in the following form was preparing, viz.

> ℞ Pulveris. craffi. radicis ipecacu-
> anhæ ʒij. aquæ bullientis ℥ viij.
> Macera in vafe fictili per horas
> quatuor. Cola liquorem, et ca-
> piat cochlearea vi. vel viij. fta-
> tim et iv. omni femi hora do-
> nec vomitus excitetur.

About one half of this infufion was given as foon as poffible, for time is as precious in this difeafe, as it is in all thofe already treated of; and if that quantity did not excite vomiting or great naufea in half an hour, four fpoonfuls more were given, and fo on till it operated upwards and downwards. It fhould be obferved, that this quantity was ordered for an adult, one half being fufficient for weakly or young people. The dofe was always eafily proportioned to the age and ftrength of the patient, as it never operated with violence, even when given in large dofes. When the fick ftrained much in vomiting, a few cups of

camomile

camomile tea or warm water were ordered;
but if they vomited with ease, no liquid was
ordered to excite it.   Chicken water, very
thin sago, or jelly of the arrow-root starch,
was given for drink and nourishment afterwards; emollient clysters were thrown up
twice or thrice a day, and sometimes an
anodyne was ordered at night.

The same ipecacuanha was infused for
four hours or all night, and the infusion repeated next morning, and frequently it was
infused a third time, and given the third
morning; but two infusions generally answered the purpose of cleansing the primæ
viæ, and from twenty-five to forty drops
of laudanum given in two ounces of the
same infusion at night, for several nights
after, very often completed the cure.   If
this infusion did not operate sufficiently by
stool, which it seldom failed to do, an ounce
and a half of the oleum ricini, made up in
the form of an emulsion with gum arabic
or the yolk of an egg, was given on the
second or third day, and the infusion with
laudanum was continued at night, or the
same

fame number of drops were added to a
ftarch clyfter.   A folution of fal cathartic
amarus in mint water, was fometimes ordered as a purgative, which anfwered very
well when it remained on the ftomach, but
as that was not often the cafe, the caftor
oil was generally preferred.   The continuance of the anodyne in the above form for
three or four nights more, together with
emollient lubricating nourifhment and
drinks, was all that was necessary in common cafes to remove the difeafe.

But when it was very violent from the
beginning, or had made great progrefs before the patient was vifited, the infufion was
given and repeated till it had operated very
well by ftool; the anodyne, as mentioned
before, was ordered every night, and the
following decoction given in the day-
time, viz.

   ℞ Pulver. craffi. corticis. Peruvian. ℥ij.
   —— Catechu vel gumi. kino. ʒij.
   Aquæ fontan. ℔iij. coque leni igne
                    ad

ad ℔ ij. cola et adde ol. cinamom
guttas iv.
Capiat ℥ ij vel ℥ iij secunda vel ter-
tia quaque hora.

When the disease did not yield to this
treatment in two or three days, some
affection of the liver, occasioning a vitiated
secretion of the bile, was suspected to be
the cause of it ; and if on examination that
viscus was found to be enlarged, hard, and
painful when pressed upon, a calomel pill
with opium was given three or four times
a day ; and when there seemed to be danger, and the case became urgent, a dram of
strong mercurial ointment was rubbed in frequently at the same time, till the gums
were affected. The pills were made up in
the following form :

℞ Calomelanos pp^{it} Ʒj
— Opii puri g^{ra} iij. in aquæ q. s.
soluti.
— Ol. cinamomi guttas iv. misce et
divide in pilulas xv
Capiat unam ter de die.

If

If frictions of mercurial ointment were used at the time thefe pills were ordered, two were fufficient in the twenty-four hours; but if the cure was trufted entirely to the pills, three or four were given in that fpace of time, till a forenefs of the gums came on, or until the difeafe was removed. During this courfe the decoction of bark was continued, to prevent a putrid tendency in the difeafe; and nourifhment of the moft lubricating kind, fometimes with wine, to fupport the ftrength of the patient, was ordered. The patient was well watched, and the mercury immediately fufpended, if it affected the gums.

The chronic hepatitis, as I have obferved in a former publication *, was almoft conftantly preceded by a purging of vitiated acrid bile, which very often brought on a dyfentery, and an abfcefs of the liver always followed, if mercury was not adminiftered early in that difeafe. Sago and panada were ufed as nourifhment for the fick; but, of

* Edin. Medical Commentaries, Decade 2d, Vol. IV. p. 317.

late

late years, the ftarch of the maranta or arrow-root of the Weft Indies has been ufed
as an emollient aliment, when made into
a jelly, for people afflicted with dyfentery,
or any other complaint of the bowels.
Wine, fugar, and fpices were added to it,
as was found neceffary, and fometimes
milk. This ftarch has been found remarkably ufeful in fuch complaints, often removing them without much affiftance from
medicine. The utility of it has been confirmed by experience, and having been
found preferable to fago, in all cafes when
both were ufed, the cultivation of it ought
to be encouraged; and if the importation of it
from our colonies, could be permitted under
certain reftrictions, it would be found much
preferable to every other aliment in diforders of the bowels, and might be employed
as fuch in our hofpitals, and in our navy
and army, and thereby prove a great faving
in the article of fago and falop, now in fuch
general ufe. The ftarch of the arum efcu-
lentum, called eddo or tanier in the Weft Indies, is equally fine and pure, and would probably be as beneficial as that of the arrow-root,
but

but it has not been so often tried. In some
cases of complaints of the bowels, this root
has been found very useful, and being more
productive in the article of starch, it could
be prepared at a much cheaper rate, and
would probably answer the same purpose *.

When a diarrhœa or lienteria followed the
dysentery, the arrow-root starch with milk
and a milk diet, seldom failed to remove it,
and restore the sick to health. It was very
often necessary to use lime-water, at the
same time, in the milk ; a pint a day taken
by degrees mixed with milk was sufficient,
and assisted in forwarding the cure. The
decoction of bark with astringents was used
for some time, when the milk diet was not
thought advisable. Sometimes a very weak
decoction of simarouba, or an infusion of
quassia root in water, was taken daily to the
quantity of a pint with good effect. The
quassia root was also infused in port wine, and

* See my paper on the comparative quantities of
starch, produced from the roots of West India plants,
used as food by the inhabitants, published in the London Medical Facts of this year.

a wine

a wine glafs full of it given three or four
times a day with advantage. Wine was never
ufed after a milk diet was begun. Flannel
was ordered to be worn over the abdomen
of thofe recovering from this difeafe, to prevent a relapfe; and it is neceffary to avoid
vegetables and acid fruits, and to pay great
attention to diet, with the fame view.

Section II.

General Remarks.

I n the treatment of the dyfentery, I have
chiefly trufted, for many years paft, to the
early ufe of ipecacuanha infufed in the manner before directed; and I can take upon
me to aver, that this practice has been attended with extraordinary fuccefs. This
may be confidered as only the renewal of
an old practice, viz. that of G. Pifo, which
I do not deny; but I think it of little confequence whether a practice is old or new,
provided that it is found by experience to be
fuccefsful. Many may probably affert, that

ipecacuanha

ipecacuanha in powder given in small doses, has been equally successful in curing the dysentery. To which I shall only reply, that I have not found this to be the case. The powder seldom purges, or so little that purgatives must be had recourse to, by which time is lost. The infusion always purges effectually, and its effects are more durable than those of the powder, and it does not fatigue or weaken the patient. It may probably impart to water its chief virtues, as the Peruvian bark does, but the preference appears to depend on its action as a gentle emetic, and a powerful purgative, at the same time, without inducing debility, by which means the disease is not allowed to gain ground nor to fix on the bowels, which a dilatory method of treatment permits it to do, and when this had been the case it too often resisted every remedy that was tried. Tartar emetic induces debility, and, on that account, should never be employed in this disease in hot climates, where the strength is so quickly exhausted, and frequently cannot be restored again by any means in our power.

I   I have

I have placed my next great dependence on mercury for the cure of this diſeaſe. It often proceeds from obſtructions or a chronic inflammation of the liver, which occaſion ſome derangement of its ſecretory or excretory organs, the cure of which can only be effected by this remedy. In general, when a diſeaſe occurs in the Weſt Indies, with ſuch ambiguous ſymptoms, that it cannot with certainty be referred to any particular claſs, ſome affection of the liver may be ſuſpected, and under ſuch circumſtances this really happened very frequently to be the caſe.

A gentle courſe of mercury for bilious complaints, even where there is no evident hardneſs of the liver, will generally prove beneficial to health in hot climates, where this viſcus is ſo often the ſeat of diſeaſes, which can only be removed by that powerful remedy, as far as we yet know.

CHAP.

CHAPTER V.

Of the Dry Belly-Ach.

Section I.

History of the Disease.

This is the most painful of all the diseases to which the inhabitants of the West Indies are liable —It begins with a sickness at the stomach, and great uneasiness about the umbilical region, which abates and returns at intervals of between ten minutes and a quarter of an hour, which become more violent every time, till at last a severe retching and vomiting comes on, which is renewed as often as the pain returns.— Equal compression over the abdomen gives a temporary relief from pain, and this circumstance, with the absence of fever and the want of a distention of the bowels, are the leading symtoms that distinguish this disease from the gastritis.

The

The bowels feem to be contracted and drawn backwards, or cramped as the patient generally expreffes it.   In the courfe of twelve or twenty-four hours the pain fometimes. becomes fo excruciating, that the poor fufferer falls into convulfions, which is always a fymptom of great danger, and in which I have known inftances of people expiring.—The torments of thofe labouring under this difeafe are beyond conception, and excite the commiferation of all who attend them, which is probably the reafon, that practitioners have fo often recourfe to opium for their relief.— A difficulty of voiding the urine comes on, and fometimes a total fuppreffion of it.— Clyfters are never retained long, and when the difeafe continues for twenty-four or thirty-fix hours with great violence, the anus is often fo much contracted, that a clyfter-pipe cannot be introduced, without great difficulty. The retching and vomiting frequently became fo violent, that even anodyne draughts were inftantly thrown up. The pulfe was always natural during the firft twelve or twenty-four hours of the difeafe,

eafe, but generally became quicker and
weaker afterwards —The heat of the body was natural at firft, but after two or
three days continuance of the difeafe, it was
much under the natural ftandard, and often
accompanied with cold fweats. Obftinate
coftivenefs always prevailed, and the common means to procure ftools were often
employed with unremitting affiduity for four
or five days to no purpofe. I have been
called to fome patients who had been in
torture for feven days without having had a
ftool ; and I vifited one the eighth day, who
had not had an evacuation by ftool all
that time, but it was then too late to afford
him any relief, for a mortification of his
bowels had taken place, and he died the
next day. The fatal termination of the above
cafe, in this way, induced me afterwards to
take eight or twelve ounces of blood from
robuft people at the commencement of the
difeafe.—Few cafes, however, occurred
that required venefection, as the people
afflicted with it had generally a pale yellow
complexion, and were more or lefs fwelled
or bloated from drinking grog, drams, or

ftrong

ftrong punch.—Only the lower orders of the white people in the Weft Indies, and the negroes, who cannot afford to drink old rum or wine, are fubject to attacks of this difeafe.

Relapfes happen very often, and fome-times bring on a degree of palfy, which is more or lefs difficult to be removed, in proportion to the preceding attacks. Al-though every patient fuffers extraordinary pain during the attacks, yet there is great variety in the degrees of violence.

It is by no means a dangerous difeafe when atended to at the beginning, but its frequent recurrence often wears out the con-ftitution, impairs the faculties of the mind, and renders a removal to a temperate cli-mate abfolutely neceffary. Or to thofe who have not the means to enable them to go to Europe or America, a total abfti-nence from fpirituous liquors fhould be ordered, and even inforced, if poffible; and drinking the hepatic or Souffriere
waters,

waters, which are to be found in moft of
thefe iflands, fhould be ftrongly recommended.

SECTION II.

Of the Cure.

WARM fomentations, applied to the abdomen, afforded only a momentary allevia-
tion of the pain, as did the femicupium,
which always weakened the patient and was
feldom repeated —Clyfters were always
given and frequently repeated, but to little
purpofe.—A blifter applied over the epigaftric region fometimes ftopped the vomiting,
by which means mild purgatives, as fal.
cathart. amarus, or an emulfion of caftor-
oil was retained on the ftomach, and being
frequently repeated, had at laft the defired
effect.—But as bliftering had not often this
good effect, and tended to increafe the fuf-
ferings of the patient, I have laid it afide
for many years paft.—Draftic purges always increafed the vomiting, and never anfwered the purpofe for which they were
given.

I 4

Two

Two grains of folid opium generally fet-
tled the ftomach and allayed the violent
fpafms in the bowels, after which an emulfion of caftor-oil, given and repeated at
proper intervals, fometimes fucceeded in
procuring ftools, although never till after
many hours perfeverance in the ufe of it.

When this gentle method of treatment
did not anfwer in the courfe of forty-eight
hours, or three days at moft, I gave fmall
dofes of calomel, fuch as three or four
grains joined to a little jalap, or extr. ca-
tharticum, twice or thrice in the twenty-
four hours, not daring, when a young practitioner, to prefcribe larger dofes for fear of
weakening and thereby hurting my patients.—When the calomel was given in fuch
fmall dofes it always affected the mouth,
and although it never failed to remove
the difeafe, even fometimes before ftools
were procured, it was attended with great
inconvenience and uneafinefs to the fick.—
The mouth, tongue, and throat were often
much fwelled, and the ptyalifm frequently
became fo very violent, notwithftanding all
                                        the

the means employed to reftrain it, that the patients not only fuffered much pain, but were often alarmed at their fituation.—I found all thofe who were attacked with this difeafe, as eafily and readily affected by mercury as fcorbutic patients are.

Although in my practice, no bad confequences ever followed a falivation, I found it fo diftreffing to the fick, and alfo fo very difagreeable to myfelf, that, after repeatedly experiencing the fame effects from this method of treatment, I was induced, when the cafe became urgent, and there appeared to be danger, to prefcribe a full dofe of calomel at once, in hopes that it would operate fo fpeedily by ftool, that the falivary glands, &c. would not be affected by it. Fifteen grains of calomel were made up into four pills, or into a bolus, with fome aromatic fpecies, and given at once; and in many cafes where the difeafe had continued five or fix days without ftools or any relief of the pain, a fcruple of calomel was made up and given in the fame way, which never failed to open the bowels in about five or

fix

fix hours, and removed the diſeaſe without bringing on a ſalivation; but the gums and mouth were generally more or leſs affected for ſeveral days after.——In ſome deſperate caſes, when called after all the uſual means had failed, and the pain and conſtipation had continued for ſeven or eight days, I have preſcribed half a dram of calomel to be made up into eight pills, which were all to be given in the courſe of four or five hours, if ſtools were not procured by the firſt ſix before the firſt period; and this bold practice was always attended with ſucceſs; which, if not attempted, the diſeaſe would have certainly proved fatal.

Nouriſhing ſoup, caudles, and mulled wine with ſpices, were neceſſary to ſupport the ſick, after the alvine diſcharge commenced, and if they became weak and faintiſh, an anodyne draught was ordered to reſtrain the immoderate purging and violent teneſmus.——Emollient clyſters were thrown up daily, ſometimes with laudanum if the teneſmus continued, and a lubricating diet, ſuch as ſago, or arrow-root——Starch
jelly

jelly with wine was ordered for feveral days
after. When the ftrength was reftored, a
table fpoonful of caftor-oil was given occafionally, if the patient was threatened with
coftivenefs.—The bark, which is fo often
prefcribed in fome form or other, to thofe
recovering from other difeafes in tropical
climates, as a tonic, and with fuch good effect
in reftoring the appetite and ftrength, has
been found hurtful after this difeafe, by
bringing on relapfes, or at leaft I thought
they were often occafioned by it, and have
therefore laid afide the ufe of it.

Palfy fucceeds a very fevere and long
continued attack of this difeafe, or proceeds
from frequent relapfes of it. To prevent
which, the cure fhould be attempted by
calomel as fpeedily as poffible, and relapfes
avoided by keeping the bowels open afterwards.

Small dofes of cathartic falts, two or
three cathartic extract pills occafionally, or
caftor-oil as mentioned before, anfwer this
laft purpofe beft.

Our

Our Souffriere waters, which are aluminous and contain much hepatic gas, have
had a good effect in preventing relapses and
curing the palsy proceeding from lead. I
have given thirty or forty drops of balsam.
peruv. on sugar, to those recovering, once
or twice a day with seeming advantage.

There can be no doubt that this is the
same disease as the colica pictonum, or De-
vonshire colic, proceeding from a solution
of lead, or from the fumes of it, by living
in painted houses; as it has been observed,
that all house-painters have the disease more
or less in the West Indies.   It has not
prevailed so much of late years as it did
fifteen or twenty years ago, owing probably
to the great attention that has been paid
to curing the rum before using it; and perhaps also to the still necks and worms being
generally now made with a mixture of tin,
instead of lead as formerly, by the hardness
of which, a solution of lead in the high proof
hot spirit, when passing through these, is
prevented; or if any particles are taken up,
they subside on the evaporation of the fiery

8   or

or volatile parts that fufpended them, in the operation of fhifting, or curing rum, as it is called *. In confirmation of this it has always been remarked, that the drinkers of new rum only are afflicted with this difeafe, or thofe who live in newly painted houfes, or fuch as are employed in painting with white lead, as was obferved before.

* The new rum runs from the ftill into five gallon cans, which is thrown into butts, from thence it is drawn off into tubs and put into puncheons, and fhifted from puncheon to puncheon every month or oftner, if wanted foon for ufe, by which its empyreumatic tafte and fmell, called haut-gout, is removed; this is what is called curing. It is fhifted only once every four or fix months when not wanted very foon. Various methods have been tried for the fpeedy curing of rum, or giving it that perfection which it attains by age and fhifting, fuch as the addition of burnt fugar or rice, and green tea; but within thefe few years paft, it has been difcovered that nothing is fo efficacious in bringing it to an early maturity, as a few handfuls of powdered charcoal thrown into each puncheon every time it is fhifted, which both improves the colour, and removes the haut-gout.

CHAP-

CHAPTER VI.

Of the Cholera Morbus.

THIS diſeaſe begins with a vomiting of thick yellow bile, and a violent diſcharge of the ſame fluid by ſtool ſoon follows.

The vomiting and purging increaſe every moment in violence, and the ſick are frequently quite exhauſted, their pulſe ſunk, and their extremities cold, before any medical aſſiſtance is called in. This often happens in the courſe of a few hours from the firſt attack.

In ſuch caſes, no time is to be loſt in adminiſtering opium, and as it will ſeldom remain on the ſtomach in a liquid form, and takes a conſiderable time to diſſolve when given in pills, it becomes neceſſary to throw up fifty or ſixty drops of laudanum in a clyſter immediately, and to give a grain of ſolid opium

at

at the same time, which muft be repeated every hour till the vomiting ceafes. When the cafe is not fo very urgent, an epithem of mint ftewed in wine, and applied warm over the pit of the ftomach, giving it the fame time two grains of opium in a pill, generally puts a ftop to the difeafe in an hour or two. Although this is by no means a dangerous difeafe, when attended to in time, yet as inftances have occurred of its proving very quickly fatal when neglected, the fpeedy adminiftration of opium ought never to be omitted. It always proceeds from a redundant, and fometimes vitiated fecretion of bile. It generally happens alfo in very hot weather; and eating large quantities of fruits and vegetables, is often the immediate caufe of it. If a yellownefs of the eyes and fkin appears after, which is fometimes the cafe, a few grains of calomel ought to be given for two or three days, when the ftrength is reftored, and a dofe of Epfom falts or caftor-oil afterwards. Directions fhould be given to the fick, to avoid eating vegetables or fruits for fome time after.

A vomiting

A vomiting and purging frequently comes on, from eating a quantity of vegetables, unripe fruits, or any thing elfe that has difagreed with the ftomach, but as little or no bile is difcharged, and this diforder feldom becomes dangerous, it is called an Indigeftion, and is cured by drinking plentifully of camomile-tea or warm water.   An anodyne draught is fometimes neceffary to allay the irritability of the ftomach, and fmall dofes of magnefia and rhubarb were generally prefcribed afterwards to reftore its tone, and to correct acidity, which always accompanies this difeafe.

CHAP-

CHAPTER VII.

Of the Tetanus, or Locked Jaw.

In my opinion this dreadful difeafe ought to be divided into two fpecies, the Idiopathic and Symptomatic, as the former often admits of a cure, whereas the latter, proceeding from a læfion of nerves or tendons, has, from my own experience, and that of all my medical acquaintance in the Weft Indies, refifted every remedy hitherto tried, having always proved fatal.

SECTION I.

Hiftory of the Difeafe.

The idiopathic tetanus proceeds from fleeping on the cold ground in the night in damp places, or from getting fuddenly wet after having been much heated, or from remaining long in wet clothes, and lying out in the cold dew. But as it happens moft fre-
K quently

quently to negroes, the caufe can very feldom be difcovered.

The fymptomatic comes on after pricks
of nails or fifh-bones in the feet, or from
fplinters of hard wood running into the feet
or hands, or from cuts of glafs bottles in
the foles of the feet or about the toes.
Alfo after pricks of fwords, and after gun-
fhot wounds in the extremities, efpecially
about the feet and ankles, after compound
fractures with fplintered bones, and after
amputations of arms, legs, fingers, or toes.
In both fpecies there is a remarkable cold-
nefs in the hands and feet, and alfo cold
fweats, but more efpecially in this laft.
This difeafe does not always, however, follow fuch punctures or læfions from accidents, or come on after operations.

I have never met with the emprofthoto-
nos in either of the fpecies. It always began
with a ftiffnefs of the mufcles of the neck
and the lower jaw. The jaws cannot be
opened more than a quarter of an inch
afunder. The head is frequently drawn
back,

back, and at the same time the jaws are
shut close. These spasms return more frequently, and with greater violence, as the
disease advances, till in forty-eight or se-
venty-two hours, if it continues so long,
the teeth are so closely shut that nothing can
be got into the mouth; the spasms become
almost incessant, every muscle of the body
is in violent action, till at last a general convulsion, in the symptomatic kind, puts a
period to life *. I knew two instances of
this disease being brought on by small fish-
bones sticking in the throat for some time,
and a negro who had it after being stung in
the glans penis when asleep, by a large
wasp called jackspaniard, in the West
Indies. They were all attacked on the
eighth or ninth day after and died.

As the trismus infantium or jaw-fall, as
it is called, never happens to infants after

---

* Although the sick had great difficulty in swallow-
ing during the spasms, they appeared to have no aversion
to water, or any other fluid, as is the case in the hydro-
phobia; nor did they slaver, or show any symptoms of
furious delirium.

the

the ninth day of their age, it may be confidered as a third fpecies of this difeafe.

SECTION II.

Of the Cure.

THE idiopathic tetanus was fometimes
cured by warm frictions, wine, opiates,
and bark. But I have fucceeded beft by
mercurial frictions, ufed every two hours all
over the neck and fpine in very large quantities, as mentioned in a former part of this
work, until the mouth was affected by it.
The mercurial ointment was feldom weighed, or the laudanum dropped in this difeafe.
Calomel was mixed with fyrup, and given
with the laudanum when the patient could
fwallow it. Wine was always given in
large quantities, and alfo nourifhing clyfters.
This method has often fucceeded in removing this direful difeafe. The cold-bath
never anfwered with me, although I have
frequently tried it. I have often wifhed to try
electricity, but never had an apparatus in
                                        perfect

perfect order till lately, since which no cases have occurred.

In the symptomatic kind, the punctures or cuts are generally healed, and after operations the stump looks well, before the disease comes on, which (when it takes place) is always on the eighth, ninth, thirteenth, or fourteenth day after the accident, or operation, as I have never known it to come on after the fifteenth.

As tetanus attacks more frequently at the first period mentioned above, than at the second ; when the first passed over I had hopes of recovery, but after the fifteenth day I never hesitated to pronounce the patient out of danger from this disease. When it unfortunately came on, I employed all the means before described for the recovery of the idiopathic kind, besides opening and scarifying the parts that had been punctured or cut, and sometimes destroying the nerve above the place, dressing the parts with mercurial ointment, and the stump with the same after operations,

K 3　　　　pouring

pouring laudanum over the lint, and giving
it by tea-spoonfuls to drink, pushing the mercurial frictions to the utmost extent, and giving plenty of wine; but all to no purpose.
The extremities were often rubbed with
mustard, Cayenne pepper, and ginger, steep-
ed in rum, &c.

As I found, from sad experience, that I
could never cure this very dreadful disease, I
thought of trying some method of preventing it.   It occurred to me, that, probably
owing to its very rapid progress, there was
not time to throw a sufficient quantity of
mercury into the system, to cure or overcome the great irritability or tendency to
violent spasmodic contractions in the mus-
cular fibres.   And as mercury seems to act
as a powerful antispasmodic in some other
diseases, I was disposed to give it a fair trial
after accidents and operations, to prevent
tetanus, knowing of no other remedy so likely
to produce that happy effect.

After wounds or punctures I therefore gave
two or three grains of calomel twice a-day, and
dressed

dreſſed the part with mercurial ointment, from the day theſe accidents happened till a gentle ſalivation came on.   And after operations I gave three grains of calomel every night with a grain and a half of opium, and three or four doſes of bark in the day-time, without regard to the ſymptomatic fever, till the mercury affected the mouth, which was generally the ſeventh or eighth day, when I gave the calomel every ſecond night only, and continued the opiate and bark till after the fifteenth day, when all was laid aſide but anodynes.   When the mercury did not begin to affect the mouth the ſeventh day, I ordered ſome mercurial ointment to be applied over a part of the ſtump, which ſeldom failed to bring it on.   Out of fifteen patients, after amputations, that were treated in this way, only one died, and he was in ſuch an irritable ſtate before the operation, that I dreaded the conſequence, and was averſe to its being performed.   He was ſeized with ſymptoms of the tetanus the eighth day, and died the ninth at night.

I do not pretend to aſſert, that the recovery

K 4   very

very of so many patients after operations, in
the West Indies, was entirely owing to this
method that I have employed for the prevention of the tetanus. In such trials nothing can
be proved with certainty. The proportion
of men who recovered by this method after
operations, is much greater, however, than
is customary in the West Indies, viz. nearly
three to one more than by the common method of treatment, as far as I have had
opportunities of observing. Its success will,
therefore, I hope, recommend it to the attention and trial of the medical gentlemen
of the navy and army in the West Indies.
It cannot prove hurtful, and from com-
paring cases in my private practice, I am
convinced of its utility. I have succeeded
in a double proportion by this treatment,
with those who had been wounded or punctured, having only lost two out of a great
number since I began it.

For many years after my arrival in the
West Indies, nearly one-fourth of the negro
children on the plantations, died of the
trismus, or jaw-fall, on the eighth or ninth
day

day after they were born. It therefore became a matter of ferious confideration with
the planters, to find out a method to prevent
this mortality among their negro children.
That the difeafe could not be cured was
foon difcovered, as not a fingle inftance of
fuch an event ever occurred. The caufe
was fuppofed to be meconium in the
bowels, or thought to proceed from the bad
inftruments that the negro midwives
ufed in cutting the navel-ftring. The
infants were purged with caftor-oil or magnefia, to remove the meconium as foon as
poffible; the midwives were furnifhed with
fharp fciffars or razors, and fhewn the proper
method of cutting and tying the navel-ftring.
But all this did not anfwer my expectations.
I obferved that the children born in large
negro-huts generally recovered; and that
white children, or thofe of free people, who
had their kitchens apart from their dwelling-
houfes, efcaped the jaw-fall; I therefore
fufpected that the fmoke from burning wood,
was the caufe of it. In confequence of this
I gave orders that no fires fhould be allowed
in the negro-houfes where the lying-in women were; which anfwered the purpofe of
preventing

preventing the difeafe, when the order was complied with; but negroes are fo fond of fire that they often lighted it up by ftealth, and thereby fruftrated my plan. 1 then recommended a lying-in-hofpital to be built on every eftate, near the negro-houfes, with a planked floor, fo that no fire could be kept in it; fince which no children, who were born in thefe hofpitals, and remained with their mothers in them for nine days, have ever been attacked with this difeafe. I wifh to recommend fuch hofpitals on every plantation in all the iflands. The negro women, however, often elude the hofpital, by concealing their pains till they cannot be moved from their own houfes; this proceeds from a love of home, or from jealoufy of their hufbands; but by perfeverance, and carrying them to the hofpital after they are delivered, all this may be overcome.

It is remarkable, that infants are never attacked with it after the ninth day of their age, as was obferved before.

The fires in the Weft Indies are made of wood, and the fmoke from them is fo ftimu-
lating

lating to the eyes, that few white people can bear it for a moment.   From the foregoing obſervations I am of opinion, that the ſmoke of wood uſed as fuel in ſmall huts where it has not a proper vent, is the cauſe of this diſeaſe among infants in ſome parts of Switzerland and France, and in the Highlands of Scotland, as well as it is in the Weſt Indies.

THE

THE
CHEMICAL ANALYSIS
AND
MEDICAL PROPERTIES
OF THE
HOT MINERAL WATERS
IN THE
ISLAND OF *DOMINICA*;

WITH SOME OBSERVATIONS ON VOLCANOS IN THE WIND-
WARD AND LEEWARD WEST INDIA ISLANDS.

THE Souffriere Waters, proceeding from
a volcano on the fouth end of this ifland,
have been ufed for various diforders with
good effects for many years paft ; but from
the beft information I have been able to
collect, no chemical analyfis of them had
ever been attempted. I had been there
on vifits to fick people frequently, but
had not time to examine thefe waters in a
chemical way ; I therefore made, at this
time, two excurfions for this exprefs purpofe.

Thefe

These mineral waters are hot, issuing from the side of a very steep ridge of mountains about two miles from the sea, forming a small rivulet which runs into it. Near to the sea-side some of the subterraneous hot waters find an outlet, and keep constantly bubbling up. This hot sulphureous water, and the water of the rivulet now become cold, may be felt at the same time. There are three craters, the uppermost of which is the largest ; there the waters boil up most violently, making a rumbling noise like distant thunder, smoking much, especially in rainy weather. In all the volcanos the water is quite black, when it issues forth from the subterraneous boilers, but soon after it turns of a pale cream colou , leaving a whitish slimy crust upon the stones below its surface. The parts of the stones above the surface of this water, are covered with a brownish or dark yellow crust, resembling ocre. The bottom and sides of the channel of the rivulet, are covered with a white earth or clay, and small porous white stones. On each side of the channel, a number of small openings, like chimnies to furnaces, were

were obferved, from which hot black vapours are conftantly iffuing. It is dangerous to approach a place where a number of
thefe fmoking openings are collected, as
the ground is hollow below, and the heat
of the fteam is equal to that of boiling
water. On the banks of the lower rivulet,
great quantities of cryftallized fulphur
are found, and a quantity of alum, fometimes pretty pure, and at other times mixed with clay or earth; it has, however,
more the appearance of burnt than common
alum.

The water has a ftrong aftringent tafte,
and a fulphureous fmell, when taken near
the fource, but it lofes the fmell after running for two or three hundred yards, when
it becomes cooler, turns white, and much
clearer. At the fource of the lower Souffriere, the water as it iffues from one of the
craters (for there are great numbers) raifed
Fahrenheit's thermometer in one minute to
205 degrees. There we found a large boiler
filled with black coloured round bullets,
from the fize of fwan-fhot to that of piftol-

§   balls,

balls, floating in the water, and in perpetual
motion from its ebullition. Thefe, when
lighted with a candle, burned away with a
beautiful purple flame, and emitted ftrong
fulphureous vapours, which tinged filver
black in a few feconds. Pure fulphur was
formed round the forceps that held thefe
balls during their combuftion; the fmall
portion of matter that remained feemed to
be earth or clay. Boiling water did not dif-
folve thefe balls thoroughly, but the water
was impregnated with all the fenfible qualities
of the Souffriere waters brought from the
fpot. About 100 yards below this crater
the thermometer, placed in the ftream of
the rivulet, rofe to 130 degrees: five gallons of water were taken from this place to
be analyfed. Where the baths now are, is
about 300 yards below the firft fource of
the water. The thermometer put into the
water at this place rofe to 106 degrees, which
upon feveral trials was found to be the medium heat there. The fource of the fecond
Souffriere is about a quarter of a mile from
the firft, and the third Souffriere is ftill higher
up, on the fide of the fame fteep mountain.
The fecond is about 200, and the third 300
yards

yards above the level of the fea. A ftrong folution of the vegetable alcali precipitated a white powder from thefe, and a large quantity of ceruffa was alfo thrown down by a tea-fpoonful of acetated lead, which we had found to be exactly the cafe with the water of the loweft Souffriere. From appearances, and the tafte of thefe upper waters, we fuppofed they contained more iron than the loweft, but upon trial with aftringents, &c. we did not find that to be the cafe. The ftreams of thefe two boiling outlets take a different courfe from the loweft, but they all unite before they reach the fea.

The land is very rugged and ftony, and the heat in the day-time here in dry weather is almoft infupportable. In our fecond excurfion, when walking in the fun about two o'clock, P. M. near the middle Souffriere, Fahrenheit's thermometer rofe to 120 degrees, and when put upon a ftone expofed to the rays of the fun, while we refted ourfelves under the fhade of a tree, it foon rofe to 138 degrees, which will appear

almoft

almost incredible, but is a fact ; and what is perhaps equally surprising, that although exposed to this extraordinary heat for several hours, we suffered no bad consequences from it *.

The vapours from these volcanos are quite black and very offensive, and occasion violent head-ach and faintness to people exposed to them for some time, but they do not appear to hurt vegetation. The upper crater makes a greater noise than the others, and throws out the steam with greater violence, but I did not observe any stones or lava thrown up when I was there ; however, I am not certain but this may be the case at times, from the appearance of the lava at some distance from the crater. There appears formerly to have been a great number of Souffrieres in this quarter of the island, which are now extinguished ; but along the sea-side hot water is found

* Mr. William Bremner, a medical gentleman of this island, accompanied me on this occasion, and assisted me in analysing the waters.

L   bubbling

bubbling from under the rocks in many places, which have the same sensible qualities as these I have described.

Chemical Analysis of the Souffriere Waters.

1st. *The Effects of Re-agents.*

Experiment 1. The vitriolic acid had no sensible effect whatever upon them.

Exp. 2.   Neither had the muriatic.

Exp. 3.   A silver coin immersed in the water was not tarnished.

Exp. 4.   The tincture of gall-nuts in strong proof spirit had little effect upon the water, after having been exposed to the air for several days.   But when it was heated, the tincture tinged it of a dark green colour, which by standing for some time became moderately black.   When a few drops of the tincture was added to a strong solution of the balls formerly mentioned, in boiling water, a very black ink was formed in a short time.

A small quantity of the aqueous infusion

fion of the rind of the pomegranate fruit,
added to the folution of the balls as above,
produced a very dark ink fit for writing in
the fpace of two hours.   A fhining purple-
coloured fcum was formed on the furface of
this folution, after the addition of the aftringent infufion.

Exp. 5. With the Pruffian alcali. A few
drops of this turned a glafs of the water of
a beautiful purple colour; and by adding
fome more, a large fediment fell to the
bottom of the glafs, which was evidently
Pruffian blue.

Exp. 6. The fixed vegetable alcali
threw down a fine whitifh coloured powder, without effervefcence

Exp. 7. Lime water produced the fame
effect as the former.

Exp. 8. The cauftic alcali occafioned
a thick greenifh cloud in the waters, which
remained fufpended in the glafs for a long
time, and after fubfiding to the bottom
turned of a very dark green colour.

Exp. 9. The volatile alcali effervefced
a little in the water, and occafioned a green
cloud in it as in the former experiment;

L 2   but

but after fubfiding it did not turn fo dark, nor was the fediment fo great. After ftanding for fome time a thick fcum formed on the top, which was evidently iron, and the clear fluid below had a very ftrong chalybeate tafte.

Exp. 10. By a few drops of acetated lead, a white powder was precipitated from a wine glafsful of the water, which had a fweetifh tafte, but feemed to be twice the quantity of ceruffa that could have been fufpended by the vinegar.

Exp. 11. Muriated barytes turned the water white, and precipitated a white heavy powder. It did the fame when added to hard water, although not in fuch a quantity; when added to pure rain water there was no fediment.

Exp. 12. Lacmus turned a wine glafs-full of the water of a light red colour—hard water was alfo turned a little red by it—but pure rain water, by adding a little of it, was turned to a beautiful blue colour.

Exp. 13 Nitrated mercury precipitated a large quantity of a beautiful orange co-loured powder—when the nitrous·acid was

afterwards

afterwards obtained very pure, the quantity
of this precipitate was not so considerable.

Exp. 14. This precipitate turned brown
when lime water was poured upon it.

Exp. 15. This last powder dissolved entirely in the muriatic acid.

Exp. 16. Acid of Sugar. This made
no change whatever upon the water, when
added to it in small or very large quantities.
—after standing for some time, the water
turned rather whiter than it was before, but
so little that it is not to be relied upon.

It is worthy of observation, perhaps, that
a solution of the sulphureous balls formerly
mentioned, in pure hot water, exhibited pre-
cisely the same chemical phenomena, with
the re-agents that the natural Souffriere waters do.

*Distillation and Evaporation of the Souffriere
Waters.*

Exp. 17. About two gallons of the water
were put into a retort with a receiver not
L 3 luted;

luted; while the diftillation was going on, black offenfive vapours came over, which tinged a filver coin quite black, in the same manner that the fteam at the fource of the Souffriere waters did. The diftilled water in the receiver was quite pure.—I had not a proper pneumato-chemical apparatus to collect and examine this gas by, but this is perhaps of lefs confequence, as it clearly appears to have been hepatic or fulphureo-hydrogenous gas.

Exp. 18. When the water in the retort turned muddy, a Florence flafk was filled with it, and being evaporated to drynefs, there remained a fine white taftelefs pow-der. Some of this powder was wafhed in high proof fpirit and dried again. Neither this powder, nor the refidue produced by the other re-agents, were inflammable.

Exp. 19. A part of this powder was mixed with water in a wine glafs, and vitri-olic acid poured upon it, which, after ftand-ing a day, began to cryftallize on the fides of the glafs, and formed a neutral falt, which was evidently alum.

Obfer-

Obfervations.

From experiments, N°. 1, 2, 3, it appears that there is no real hepar fulphuris in thefe mineral waters; but from exp. 17, it is plain and evident that they abound with hepatic gas, or, according to Monf. de Fourcroy, being only impregnated with that gas, they may be termed hepatized thermal waters.

Exp. 4. And more particularly exp. 5. fhew that they contain iron fufpended probably by the vitriolic acid, as appears from expts. 11 and 12. Heat feems alfo to have fome power in keeping the iron diffolved, as great quantities of ocre were depofited on the ftones in the rivulet, when the water became perfectly cold. They feemed then to poffefs only a weak impregnation of that metal.

Exp. 6, 7, 8, 9, 10, prove that an earth is fufpended by an acid, and the fynthetic exp. 19 proves that acid to be the vitriolic, and that earth to be clay, of which there

L 4 · is

is more than sufficient to saturate the acid.
The yellow precipitate produced by the nitrated mercury, is not so easily accounted
for.—The hot waters at Bath produce the
same phenomenon with this solution of mercury, according to Dr. Charleton's analysis ;
but it does not appear to proceed from an
alcaline. principle in our Souffriere waters,
as he asserts it does in the waters at Bath,
as is clearly proved from exp. 16. the acid
of sugar being the best test for discovering
calcareous earth, or any other alcaline earth.

It appears from exp. 15. that this precipitate was Turpeth mineral, as it dissolved
entirely in the muriatic acid, from which,
probably, corrosive sublimate might have
been obtained, if there had been a sufficient quantity collected to have tried the
experiment.   These waters are strongly
impregnated with alum, with excess of a fine
white clay, pure hepatic gas, and vitriolat-
ed iron; from which they may be termed
thermal, aluminous, hepatized waters, with
a portion of iron suspended in them.

All

All round the volcano this hepatic gas is poured forth from innumerable openings, like small chimnies, on the edges or sides of which pure flowers of sulphur are formed. This is a beautiful phenomenon, which probably arises from the vital air of the atmosphere decomposing this hepatic gas, and thereby depositing its sulphureous part—drops of pure water were found hanging from these openings.

Medical properties of the Souffriere waters.

BATHS and accommodations for sick people were built many years ago; which having been neglected for some time past, are now almost decayed. The water at the baths, as I observed before, rose Fahrenheit's thermometer to 106 degrees, but there is a bath where the water is received and allowed to cool to that degree of heat which is directed by the physician. The water is generally drank at about natural heat or 98°, but sometimes it is used when quite cold. The general effects of it are to promote perspiration when drank warm, and when cold it

appears

appears to act as a tonic. The itch, scorbutic, and herpetic eruptions, and all cutaneous diseases are relieved, and most commonly removed entirely, by bathing twice a day for some time in the water, allowed to cool to the degree of natural heat. Rheumatic disorders of the chronic kind were greatly relieved, and sometimes cured by bathing. Anchylosis, rigid tendons, and stiffness of the small joints, when they did not proceed from a siphylitic cause, were cured by the douche, bathing, and drinking the waters. They have been employed very frequently in paralytic disorders, and in those proceeding from the dry belly-ach, which is occasioned by lead, as was observed before, they were very efficacious, seldom failing to effect a perfect cure.

In complaints of the stomach and bowels proceeding from the fumes of lead, in giddiness of the head, trembling of the limbs, tingling at the ends of the fingers, and other nervous affections, so common among housepainters, or among other people, occasioned by their living in newly painted houses, or drinking much new rum; the Souffriere

waters

waters drank lukewarm, three or four times a-day, and bathing in them once or twice a-day, contributed very much to alleviate, and fometimes removed them entirely. A good diet and exercife were ufed at the fame time; but to reftore the ftrength, and thereby complete the cure, the cold fea-bath was generally neceffary. In the hemiplegia, or lefs violent paralytic affections, proceeding from an apoplectic attack, they were not found to be fo beneficial, although drank cold, and the bath ufed nearly cold. In one inftance they proved evidently hurtful, but the bath was ufed hot, and the bad effects proceeded, probably, from that circumftance. In general, they may be employed for the fame complaints for which the Bath waters are ordered, and with equal advantage.

General Obfervations.

NEAR the middle of this Ifland on the top of a high mountain, there is a much larger volcano ftill burning, than that now defcribed. It forms a hollow refembling a punch bowl, and occupies a fpace of ground
equal

equal to 12 or 15 acres. A small river of hot Souffriere water issues from this volcano, having the same sensible qualities as those which have been analysed. I have seen and tasted the water near the sea-side, but the description of the place is from the information of people who have been on the spot, as a journey to a part of the Island so difficult of access was too fatiguing for me to undertake. In all our Windward and Leeward Islands, there have been similar volcanos, most of which are now burnt out; but their remains are easily discovered by the hot water that is poured forth at some distance from them, and by exploring the mountains, as Morne Agrou was in Saint Vincent, by Mr. Anderson, who has given a very accurate and ingenious description of a large volcanic crater in that mountain, in the Philosophical Transactions. There are hot waters in the Islands of Saint Christopher' and Nevis, but the volcanos there have been extinguished long ago. Evident marks of different craters are to be seen in the mountains there, and also in the Island of St. Eustatius. Many small Souffrieres are burnt out in this Island, and also

in

in Martinico and Guadalqupe.   There are several volcanos still burning in these Islands, the waters of which resemble ours in every respect, and are employed for the cure of the same diseases.

In the Island of Guadaloupe particularly, there is a very large volcano, which throws out great quantities of lava, and can be seen smoking at a great distance.

The difference in the qualities of the hot waters of these Islands, arises from the strata of earth and minerals that they pass over. In some there is probably a bed of clay, or calcareous or magnesian earth and iron ore. In our Island it passes through argillaceous earth, and this seems to be the case in all the Islands that I have visited, for they all abound with clay, and a variety of pottery is made in every one of them.   All have pyrites, black sand, that is attracted by the magnet, or iron ore in some form or other. Sulphur is also always found near and in the burning volcanos, and all pour forth the same hepatic gas.   Large quantities of sulphur

phur are found in banks all round the craters, after the fubterraneous fires are extinguifhed.   It appears very evidently, that
volcanos have been burning in all the Windward and Leeward Weft India Iflands, at
fome period of time;   and that in thofe
fituated lowest, the fire has burnt out
firft, and continued to burn longeft in the
higheft or moft mountainous.   In the low
Iflands of Barbadoes, Antigua, Nevis, and
Marigalante, they have been extinguifhed
long ago, but continue to burn in many
places in Martinico, Guadaloupe, and in this
Ifland, which is the moft broken and the
moft elevated of them all.

Volcanic ftones are found on the ridges
or tops of mountains in all thefe Iflands,
either in a vitrified ftate, or in lava of a
white or gray colour, being very light and
porous, having black and fhining fpots in-
terfperfed in them, which being cut or dug
out, appeared to be bits of fehorl.   Some of
thefe ftones are of a more compact texture,
and being capable of refifting the greateft
                                        heat

heat without cracking or flying, are called
fire-ftones, and are ufed for hanging or
building coppers and ftills for boiling of fugar and diftilling of rum.   The tufa or lava
found near the openings of old volcanos, is
very light and fpungy, generally of a pale
white or reddifh colour, and in places where
it has been long expofed to the air, it is
mouldered into a fort of foft gravel.   Coral
rocks are found at a great height above the
furface of the fea, all round the fea coaft of
thefe Iflands, fometimes in ftrata covered
with earth, but more frequently in large
maffes; from which, by burning, lime is
made.   Coral rocks are always formed at
the bottom of the fea, by the petrifaction,
or incruftation of coral, fea-weeds, and other
fubmarine plants.

Earthquakes have not been fo frequent
nor fo violent for thefe twenty years paft, as
they were formerly, according to the ac-
counts given of them by the oldeft inhabitants.

How

How thefe fubterraneous fires are gene-
rated in the bowels of the earth, is a queftion of very difficult folution; the difcuffion
of which I fhall not prefume to enter upon
at prefent, although I may make fome attempt of that kind, when I am more at
leifure.

F I N I S.

E R R A T A.

In page 18, dele " violent."
   D° 115, *for* " which" *infert* " and."
   D° 118, *inftead of* " the" *infert* " its."

APPENDIX.

EXPERIMENTS

ON THE

CINCHONA BRACHYCARPA.

By Mr. BRANDE,

APOTHECARY TO THE QUEEN.

1ft. WATER and fpirit diftilled from it, became flightly impregnated with a peculiar aromatic flavor, not difco-verable in any other preparation.

2d. The decoction ʒij to ℥vj of water boiled to ℥iv is of a deep color, clear, and poffeffes the whole flavor of the bark; on cooling it becomes turbid, and depofits a powdery fediment, but lefs in quantity than the common Peruvian, the yellow, or an-gaftura bark, which, as in thefe, is again nearly foluble by the addition of the vege-table or mineral acids, &c. *

3d. The infufion ʒij to ℥iv of boiling

---

* I had not obferved the importance attached by Dr. Relph, to the property poffeffed by the decoction of the yellow bark, of remaining found a much longer time than either that of the common or red bark, till within a few days of the above being fent to the prefs, therefore had not time to compare the cinchona brachyocarpa, with it in this refpect. *Vide his Inquiry, &c. p.* 133.

water,

water, appeared equally ftrong as the decoction, and remained clear.

4th. On ʒij were poured ʒiv of cold water,
and frequently fhaken during twelve hours,
then ftrained; this infufion appeared nearly
of equal ftrength with the above; three frefh
portions of water were then poured upon
the bark, and being ftrained were mixed
together. Two ounces of rectified fpirit
were added to the refiduum, which, after
digefting eighteen hours, had extracted
very little tafte or color.

5th. The tincture one ounce to four of
rectified fpirit (which was afterwards ufed
for the refinous extract) was deep colored,
but with little tafte.

6th. Proof fpirit is a good menftruum;
but fpirit diluted with three or four parts
of water is the beft.

7th. Solutions of pure, and carbonate of
potafh, extracted deep tinctures, but lefs fo
than thofe of ammonia.

8th. Dilute fulphuric acid extracted a
very flight tafte and color.

9th. Diftilled vinegar diffolved but little.

10th. Sp. ætheris vitriol extracted very
little.

11th.

11th. Sp. ætheris nitros. is a somewhat better; by no means a good menstruum.

12th. Lime-water made an infusion of a very deep color, but without much taste.

13th. One drachm rubbed with 30 grains of lime, yielded ammonia scarcely sufficient to be smelt, but enough very sensibly to whiten the fumes of muriatic acid; on this mixture were poured two ounces of cold water; the infusion, after standing 24 hours, was of a deep red color, without much flavor.

14th. One drachm was rubbed with an equal quantity of pure magnesia; the same was done with carbonate of magnesia; and four ounces of boiling water gradually added to each : having stood 12 hours, the former appeared somewhat stronger, the latter perhaps weaker than a common infusion; the former gave the darkest precipitate with solution of iron, but not more so than the common decoction.

15th. Compared with equal quantities of infusions of the common, the yellow bark, and galls, it appeared to contain evidently more astringent matter than the two former; less than the latter.

16th. The cold infusion, No. 4. yielded
M 2 on

on evaporation 53 grains of a clear, bitter, dry extract.

17th. Two ounces gave, by pouring boiling water over them in a flannel bag, as long as it received either taste, or color. and gentle evaporation, ʒ vij. gr. v. of a pilular extract.

18th. The tincture (No. 5.) yielded on evaporation 69 grains of a hard extract, nearly soluble by trituration in hot or cold water, the residuum of bark was boiled in a quart of water to three ounces, strained and evaporated to the consistence of honey ; to which was added the resinous part, previously dissolved in a little alcohol, and the evaporation continued nearly to dryness, when the whole weighed four drachms five grains.

19th. One ounce distilled alone in an earthen retort, produced pyrolygnous acid, empyreumatic oil, and other gasses, the properties and quantities of which I was prevented from ascertaining, by an accident which befel my apparatus. The residuum burnt in the retort to a coal weighed ʒij. gr. viij.

20th. On the 128 grains of coal in the last experiment, were poured eight ounces of boiling distilled water; after standing a short time

time the folution was filtered; to different portions of which were added feveral tefts, of thefe exotic acid, nitrate of filver, and muriate of barytis; each formed a milky precipitate.

21ft. On the coal left behind was poured fome dilute fulphuric acid; this paffed through a filter, gave pruffiate of iron on the addition of pruffiate of potafh, but difcovered nothing elfe to any teft made ufe of.

22d. From the fame quantity of coal obtained, as in No. 19. by the addition of diftilled water, filtration, and evaporation, I obtained fix grains of the following falts: fulphate of potafh, muriate of potafh, carbonate of potafh and lime, perhaps pure. The iron alfo in No. 21. was in very fmall quantity.

The following Table will fhew the quantity of foluble or extractive matter obtained from this and the other barks now in general ufe, for which I am indebted chiefly to Mr. Babington's Letter in Dr. Relph's Treatife on the Yellow Bark; fome allowance is perhaps to be made for the different confiftence to which each extract may have been evaporated. I muft alfo remark, the quantity of extract I obtain from common Peruvian bark, either aqueous or fpirituous, is conftantly greater than that mentioned by

Mr.

Mr. Babington, generally amounting from three to four ounces out of twelve.

From	By cold water.	By boiling water.	By rectified spirit.	By spirit and water.
Cinchona Brachycarpa was obtained.	ʒij. ℈3 gr.	ʒji. ʒvij. gr. v.	ʒj. ʒi. gr. ix.	ʒj. ʒiv. gr. v.
Angustura bark.	ʒiv. ʒvi. ℈ij.	℔j. ʒvi. ʒiv. ℈ij.	ʒiv. ʒiv.	℔j. ʒvij. ℈ij.
Yellow Peruvian bark.	℔v. ʒxv.	℔x. ℔iv. ʒij.	ʒxij. ʒxiij.	℔j. ʒiv.
Red bark.	—	℔x. ℔iv. ʒi.	—	℔j. ʒij. ⁶⁄₈.
Common Peruvian bark.	—	℔x. ℔ij. ʒix.	—	℔j. ʒij. ³⁄₄.

It is prefumed that every pound mentioned here, is that of the Apothecary's or Troy weight.

To

To afcertain its power of preventing and
correcting putrefaction, feveral experiments
were made with a great variety of fub-
ftances, of which it will be fufficient to obferve, that the cinchona brachycarpa was generally found nearly equal to any as a pre-
ventive, inferior to the anguftura as a cor-
rective of putrefcence; it coincided very
much with the yellow bark, both of which
poffefs, in this refpect, qualities fomewhat
fuperior to the common Peruvian.

Having afcertained thus much, I fhall
only infert the following experiment :

Seven phials, each containing ʒij. of frefh
fheep gall and ʒij. of water were numbered;
to the firft was added 10 gr. of fine powdered cinchon. brachyc. to the fecond, 10
gr. of anguftura; to the third, the fame of
yellow bark; to the fourth, an equal quantity of frefh burnt charcoal, and three were
left without any addition, as ftandards or for
future ufe.——Thefe were placed together by
the fide of a fire, where the medium of heat
for 16 or 18 hours of the 24, was about
96 degrees of Fahrenheit's thermometer,
and frequently fhaken.——At the expiration
of 20 hours, 1, 2, 3, 4 were quite fweet;

5, 6, 7 fmelt very bad; to No. 5, 10 grains of cinch. brach. were added; to No. 6, of anguftura; to No. 7, of yellow bark, the fame quantities.

44 Hour—all were fweet.

56 Hours—No. 3, 4, and 6 were becoming offenfive, the reft were fweet.

68 Hours—No. 2 and 6 remained fweet, the others all fmelt very offenfive—No. 4, confiderably the worft, to which were added fix grains of the fubftance each already contained.

24 Hours had elapfed before they were examined again, when 1 and 2 were fweet, 3 fmelt a little, 4 was very bad, 6 remained perfectly fweet, 5 and 7 were again becoming putrid, but no other alteration appeared to have taken place after feveral hours.

Printed in the United States
By Bookmasters